Hospital Efficiency and Public Policy

Harry I. Greenfield

Published in cooperation with
the Center for Policy Research, Inc.

The Praeger Special Studies program—utilizing the most modern and efficient book production techniques and a selective worldwide distribution network—makes available to the academic, government, and business communities significant, timely research in U.S. and international economic, social, and political development.

Hospital Efficiency and Public Policy

PRAEGER SPECIAL STUDIES IN U.S. ECONOMIC, SOCIAL, AND POLITICAL ISSUES

Praeger Publishers   New York   Washington   London

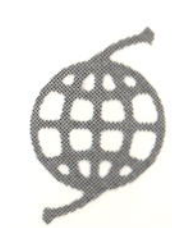

Library of Congress Cataloging in Publication Data

Greenfield, Harry I   1922-
    Hospital efficiency and public policy.

    (Praeger special studies in U.S. economic,
social, and political issues)
    Bibliography: p.
    1. Hospitals—Administration. 2. Medical
economics. 3. Hospital utilization. I. Title.
[DNLM: 1. Economics, Hospital—U.S.
2. Hospital administration—U.S. WX 157 G796h
1973]
RA971.3.G7 1973   362.1'1   72-14205

PRAEGER PUBLISHERS
111 Fourth Avenue, New York, N.Y. 10003, U.S.A.
5, Cromwell Place, London S.W.7, England

Published in the United States of America in 1973
by Praeger Publishers, Inc.

Printed in the United States of America

The tired word "crisis" takes on a sad new vitality when applied to American hospitals. Costs are skyrocketting so rapidly that even the most affluent of nations are hard put to fuel the system. This means that those services allotted by the pocketbook are increasingly becoming the title of the very rich, and those which are publicly financed must compete unfavorably with scores of other services whose costs also rise, if not as drastically. Most basically, more costs per unit means that whatever the budget there will be fewer units and less service.

Surprisingly, economists have not seen fit to dedicate their talents to the understanding and alleviation of this problem. Like many other social scientists, often more so, economists are concerned with basic research, model building, and mathematical exercises. It is a widely held belief that these are the shortest and best ways to prepare the ground for applied solutions. I doubt it. I suggest that an empirical study of the use of econometrics in most applied fields, from development to health economics, would show that the models are of limited value, and that much additional applied work must be used, in conjunction with, or instead of abstract models before we make progress.

Greenfield's study is an attempt to advance this field. Because he cannot stand on a pile of accumulated knowledge or draw on a rich body of work conducted by peers, much of this work must be viewed as an effort to break new ground, to seek new measurements in an area in which data are lacking and indicators elusive, and to find ways of getting a grip on a topic which heretofore has so often escaped the grasp of economists.

Greenfield's, like all good policy-relevant work, must also straddle two disciplines. Hence this book will be of interest not only to the applied economist but also to the student of administration. It concerns not only hospitals as individual organizations but also as complexes—as hospital systems—organizations in which the cost crisis might have to be faced.

Greenfield moves beyond the basic unit of health care to the study of health care systems, from microeconomics to macroeconomics. There is good reason to believe that both the opportunites and the curbs of more effective public policy rest on this more encompassing level. Rather than seeking to deal directly with the decisions of millions of patients and hundreds of thousands of doctors and other health professionals in thousands of hospitals we must evolve effective procedures that can affect the total health environment.

Also, as our society is a pluralistic one, even if government ownership or control did "work," surely it is not a basis for the solution of our many and varied health problems. Greater public guidance (Greenfield calls it "suspension") is clearly the direction toward which a solution might evolve.

Thus this volume, like several other books resulting from work carried out under the auspices of the Center for Policy Research, indicates how the lenses of scholarship may be focused on policy problems. We promise no easy, rapid solutions; the world is too complex for that. We promise genuine concern with the world rather than detachment, an honest attempt to bridge theory and research with the world of policy-making.

Amitai Etzioni
Director

The field of scholarship, like so many others, operates on a double-entry bookkeeping principle. No sooner is a book completed than debts are incurred. Unlike other cases in which debt repayment entails costs, however, here it is laden with pleasurable utilities.

It is a pleasure, then, to express my indebtedness to Amitai Etzioni, Director of the Center for Policy Research, who provided me with the opportunity to do the research and writing for the present study. I am also grateful to my colleagues at the Center who provided a stimulating interdisciplinary milieu, some of the benefits of which, I hope, appear in these pages. I have also been fortunate in having had access to the advice of hospital administrators, Blue Cross executives, the research departments of the American Medical and American Hospital associations, and of various state health departments.

This work, part of a larger study of cost consciousness in the health field, was funded by the Department of Health, Education and Welfare, National Institutes of Health, Grant Number 3 RO1 HS00197-02S1.

None of the above organizations or individuals is implicated in the errors of fact or interpretation that might have been committed by the author in the manuscript.

Page

LIST OF TABLES

The 1971 Economic Report of the President* identified three major problems facing national programs in the health field: the uneven distribution of health services arising from income disparities and geographic barriers; disequilibrium stemming from increased effective demand (in large part via government funds) and relatively inelastic supply (largely manpower deficiencies and organizational inflexibility); and inefficient utilization of the resources (inputs) devoted to health care. All three are, of course, intimately related. Increased efficiency in resource utilization, in terms of productivity increases, for instance, can help narrow the gap between supply and demand in a given area and, moreover, can help lower barriers to accessibility based on income and geography—in the former case by restraining inflation and perhaps reducing unit prices, in the latter by utilizing state-of-the-art multiphasic screening, computer analysis, and remote terminal diagnosis by specialists.

The focus of the present study is on the third problem cited in the Economic Report—efficiency. More specifically, we are concerned with efficient utilization of resources in the hospital, though obviously one must also deal with the relationships among hospitals and with those between hospitals and other types of health facilities to present a more comprehensive analysis.

In the following chapters we shall attempt to define efficiency in the hospital context, to analyze major promoting and inhibiting factors affecting efficiency, to evaluate major empirical studies of hospital efficiency, to present current data from a sample of hospitals that illustrate facets of efficiency, and to point up avenues for promoting efficiency that appear to be the most fruitful to pursue.

There is obviously a broad interface here between economic analysis and organization theory; the focus of this work is on the former. It is hoped that those who approach the health field via the latter route will be able to utilize economic insights in the present study.

---

*Economic Report of the President, February 1971, Washington, D.C. p. 137.

Hospital Efficiency and Public Policy

The belief is widespread among all segments of the population that hospitals are inefficient organizations. This belief is reinforced with each hospital bill issued to a patient and with the quarterly reports of the apparently uncontrollable rise in the hospital daily charges component of the medical care price index. If the prices of all goods and services rose at approximately the same rates, hospital prices would not be singled out as a particular target of attack. Hospital prices, however, are rising at a far greater rate than are goods or services or of medical care costs as a whole. Hospitals, in short, have priced themselves into the public eye. For example, using 1967 as "100," the Consumer Price Index (CPI) rose from 95.4 in December 1965 to 119.1 in December 1970, an increase of 23.7 index points. The medical care component of the CPI rose from 90.5 to 124.2, a rise of 33.7 index points. Hospital daily service charges rose from 78.5 to 152.0, a 73.5 increase in index points.[1] Another way of looking at these relationships is shown in Table 1.1.

Compared with the average annual change in prices of all goods and services (more correctly all of those included in the CPI), hospital daily services charges increased 3.3 times faster in 1966, 6.6 times faster in 1967, 3.1 times faster in 1968, 2.4 times faster in 1969, and 2.1 times faster in 1970. All of these indexes, however, are stated in relative terms and do not reflect the full impact of a hospital bill. In New York City, for example, charges of $150 per day are common and when multiplied by an average stay of about eight days the hospital charges alone, exclusive of physician fees and special services, reach $1200.*

---

*Sen. Abraham Ribicoff cites forecasts of $1,000 per day by 1980; cf. The New York Times, May 27, 1970. See also The New York

TABLE 1.1

Percentage Changes in Consumer Price
Index and Selected Medical Care
Components, 1966-70

	Average annual percent increase				
	1966	1967	1968	1969	1970
CPI, all items	2.9	2.9	4.2	5.4	5.9
Medical care, total	4.4	7.1	6.1	6.9	6.3
Physicians' fees	5.8	7.1	5.6	6.9	7.5
Dentists' fees	3.3	5.0	5.5	7.0	5.8
Hospital daily service charges	9.7	19.0	13.2	13.0	12.5
Drugs and prescriptions	.3	-.5	.2	1.1	2.3

<u>Source</u>: Research and Statistics Note, U.S. Dep't. of H.E.W., Social Security Administration, March 23, 1971, p. 6.

Over a time span of almost four decades, separating out population changes and changes in technology and utilization factors, the pure price increase component still predominates, as the following data show:

In Table 1.2 column 1 utilizes the same component of the Common Price Index as in Table 1.1. Column 2 represents hospital reported expenses. Column 3 shows consumer spending divided by total inpatient days. The bottom panel indicates that in the shorter (post-Medicare or post-Medicaid) period from 1966-68, the pure inflationary component is even more prominent.

If, as Gardner Ackley has stated,* inflation is now "clearly an endemic problem in the Atlantic world" (why the parochialism?), it would appear that hyperinflation is endemic to the world of health services.

We shall look further into the questions of hospital costs and charges in a subsequent chapter. Our present aim in discussing them is to point up the problem. For the moment our interest is focused on the nature of the hospital as a productive unit, as an economic entity with associated inputs and outputs in the hope that by gaining insights into its structure, operations, and functions we might move

---

<u>Times</u>, November 3, 1971 where it is reported that per diem rates rose from $30 in 1955 to $150 currently.

*<u>The New York Times</u>, July 26, 1971.

closer to an understanding of the central questions of efficiency and
the mirror-image costs, posed at the outset.

THE HOSPITAL AS A FIRM

A serious communications gap exists among researchers in
the health field. On one side we find those trained in medical and
public health fields, on the other recent "interlopers" from the social
sciences. This is not to suggest that there are no problems on both
sides but simply to note that the larger gulf occurs between medical
and nonmedical groups. And one of the most important reasons for
this mutual misunderstanding arises from the analogy that every
economist makes on first contact with the health field—the hospital
as a firm. We shall elaborate on this theme, attempting to indicate
its heuristic value in the analysis of hospital efficiency.

Resistance to the use of the "firm" concept stems mainly from
the general equation in our economy between firms and profit-seeking.

TABLE 1.2

Sources of Increase in Hospital Expenditures

Factor	Daily service charge, CPI (1)	Expense per patient day (2)	Expenditures per inpatient-day (3)
Long run (1929-68)			
Total	100.0	100.0	100.0
Price	60.8	72.4	73.2
Population	13.4	13.3	13.4
All other	25.8	14.3	13.4
Short run (1966-68)			
Total	100.0	100.0	100.0
Price	94.2	78.6	78.4
Population	6.4	6.5	6.6
All other	-0.6	14.9	15.0

Source: Adapted from "Sources of Increase in Selected Medical
Expenditures, 1929-1969," Social Security Administration, Staff Paper
No. 4, April 1970, p. 26.

Most firms are, in fact, business entities that seek to generate profits
from their production activities. By definition a firm is a productive
unit organized by an entrepreneur or group of entrepreneurs for the
express purpose of realizing a profit on a short or long run time
horizon. Various inputs are hired and set to work producing an output that might be either a tangible good or an intangible service,
or both. Entrepreneurs seek to maximize profits or to minimize
losses. Although some critics questions the maximizing assumption
for larger corporations, this debate is not germane to the present
discussion.

In recent years, however, increasing attention is being paid to
the large and growing sector of our economy that consists of firms
that are not profit-making.[2] This sector is composed of such entities
as government units, philanthropic groups, educational organizations,
non-profit research agencies, sectarian organizations, and a large
segment of the health care "industry." As one writer put it, "Since
decisions made by non-profit institutions affect the allocation of
[society's] resources, it is important that their decision-making
powers be understood."[3]

The boundaries of the "health care industry," like those of every
other industry, are not fixed but depend for their definition on the
observer, the pace and nature of technological change, and the purposes
of the analysis. The industry falls basically into the services category
of the goods-services dichotomy and central to the provision of health
services is the hospital.[4] Returning to the firm analogy, the question
arises: What is the hospital counterpart to the firm's entrepreneurial
function? Before attempting to answer this question one must note
that in earlier stages of development both ownership and control
resided in the entrepreneur. With the growth of large corporate
entities (as noted in the 1930s by Berle and Means and more recently
by Galbraith) a bifurcation has developed. Owners—in some cases
millions of shareholders—exercise little or no control, the latter
function having been taken over by what Galbraith has termed the
technostructure, that is to say the group that brings specialized
knowledge, talent, or experience to group decision-making.[5] Direct
application of these ideas to the hospital is somewhat complicated
by the threefold division of ownership and/or control that prevails,
viz. voluntary nonprofit, (sometimes called "community"), governmental, and proprietary institutions. Table 1.3 provides an overview
of the hospital field in terms of facilities and beds under the three
control types and by whether the institution caters primarily to short-
term or long-term patients (i.e. where over 50 percent of all patients
admitted have a stay of more or less than 30 days).[6] As may be seen,
88 percent of all hospitals are of the short-term variety and unless
otherwise noted our discussion refers primarily to these.

TABLE 1.3

Hospitals and Beds in the United States
by Ownership, 1969

	Hospitals	Beds
U.S. Total	7,144	1,650,000
Short term	6,272	926,581
Short term as percent of total	88	56
Short Term		
Nongovernmental nonprofit	3,456	581,959
Nongovernmental for-profit	799	50,826
Governmental (federal, state & local)	2,017	293,796
Nongovernmental nonprofit as percent of short term	55	63
Nongovernmental for-profit as percent of short term	13	5
Governmental (federal, state & local) as percent of short term	32	32

Source: Hospitals - Guide Issue, Part two, Tables 1 and 2,
August 1, 1970.

Quantitatively, the nongovernmental nonprofit (voluntary) hospitals
are the most important with 55 percent of the hospitals, with 63 percent of the beds under this control type. Governmental units rank
second, proprietary hospitals third. If we use the nonprofit criterion
and combine voluntary and governmental units, we note that 87 percent of the short-term hospitals and 95 percent of the beds are under
not-for-profit auspices—a fact that bears significantly on both our
previous and subsequent discussions. In voluntary hospitals, for
instance, unlike the case of business firms, the managerial problem
did not arise, as mentioned earlier, from the divorce of ownership
from control since ownership resides in a "community" or in a nonprofit philanthropic or religious association. In one sense, therefore—
with the exception of proprietary facilities, there was never an
"entrepreneur" in whom the dual functions resided. Typically, the

organizational structure of the hospital is tricapitate:* the board of
trustees (representing the "owners"), the medical staff (which functions
as the technostructure), and the administrator (whose role is comparable to that of the top management of a business firm). It is
important to note, however, that when conflicts among the groups
arise, ". . . the board [of trustees] almost invariably decides in favor
of the medical staff."[7]

In economic terms the hospital may be thought of as a plant
whose inputs consist of labor of various grades and skills, fixed capital
(land, buildings, beds, and equipment) and circulating capital (food,
bandages, bedding, drugs, etc.) with their associated costs. It is the
function primarily of the administrative and medical staffs so to
combine these inputs that they achieve a maximum impact in terms
of improved functioning on "the consumer" of the product—the patient.
In proprietary institutions the administrator or owners would seek
to keep the costs of production at a minimum and attempt to obtain
maximum revenues so that the rate of profit per capital invested would
be maximized. The management of nonprofit hospitals, governmental
or other, however, is not similarly motivated since there are no
"owners" who seek to maximize the return on their investment.**
The business model of the firm which is based on short or long run
profit maximization (or even 'satisficing behavior') does not apply or
requires serious modification. Newhouse has suggested that there
are two elements in the nonprofit decision maker's maximand: the
quantity of service and the quality of service rendered.[8] These vari-
ables, of course, are not completely independent of each other in that
tradeoffs are certainly possible between them. In the pursuit of these
goals, or more usually, of a goal that is a compromise, voluntary
hospitals have traditionally incurred deficits in the annual summary
of their operations. Although deficits are usual, hence expected, it
might nevertheless be either a conscious or unconscious goal of the
administration to minimize the deficit or even to maximize a surplus—
a result of operating revenues exceeding costs. We shall discuss
these matters further in considering pricing and output decisions in
a later chapter.

The central concern of this study is not the development of a
general organizational theory of voluntary hospitals. If we proceed

---

*Quadrupartite, if nurses are considered separately from the
medical staff.

**It might be argued that in many cases, particularly in rural
communities, the voluntary hospital's actions may be explained in
large part by the desire of referring physicians to maximize their
incomes.

on the assumption that the goal of short run or long run profit maximization does not hold for nonprofit hospitals, however, we are led
to consideration of other goals that might help explain the actions of
hospital decision-makers. This knowledge is essential if realistic
policy recommendations are to be formulated and implemented.

Although there are conflicts of interest among the control
groups—trustees, medical staff, and administrator—one goal common
to all is "prestige." A hospital's prestige is a function of its size,
the variety of state-of-the-art facilities and services it offers, the
fame and ability of the physicians affiliated with it in one way or another, its own affiliation with a medical school, the quality of its
research, its status as a teaching hospital, and perhaps the degree
of control it exercises over other institutions. Some of these goals
are subsumed and concretized in O. E. Williamson's formulation of
the behavior of firms, to wit: ". . . [M]anagers are held to operate
the firm so as to maximize a utility function that has as principal
components (1) salaries, (2) staff, (3) discretionary spending for
investments and (4) management slack absorbed as cost."[9] (It need
hardly be added that long-term survival of the hospital is also a goal
common to the "organizational coalition."[10]) Williamson's concept of
organizational or managerial slack is interesting. He defines it as
"the difference between the payments required to maintain the organization and the resources obtained from the environment by the coalition,"[11] in economic terms—a kind of coalition economic rent. This
concept is, of course, central to the notion of efficiency. In terms of
a comparative analysis of efficiency in profit and nonprofit enterprises
the determination of the degree of slack would appear to be a major
determinant of the differential—if one exists.

We have touched so far on the notion of inputs to the hospital
and the goals of management in utilizing those inputs to produce an
"output," defined earlier as a patient who hopefully has benefited,
to some not easily quantifiable degree, from his hospital stay. Since
the measurement of improved patient functioning is not yet standard
procedure in the evaluation of hospital output, it is customary to use
surrogates to measure the level of hospital activities, e.g. admissions,
discharges, days of patient care, number of cases treated, occupancy
rates, and out-patient and emergency room visits. These output
measures will be discussed in connection with our analysis of productivity measures.*

---

*Strictly speaking, hospitals may also produce other outputs,
such as education of interns, residents, nurses, and other personnel;
research; social services; and community education. In voluntary
hospitals greatest emphasis would be placed on the patient with other

As implied above, economic analyses of the not-for-profit sector
and of particular nonprofit firms are not extensive. We have shown
further that in the case of hospitals we are dealing primarily with a
nonprofit milieu and from the point of view of the institutions themselves, with nonmarket incentives. Until relatively recently, and
even now on a very preliminary basis, there has been no federal
planning or coordination in the hospital area. There has been a
somewhat greater effort at planning on a state level with predictably
great variations among the states and little planning even on a city or
county level. The result has been a haphazard proliferation of hospitals
and other types of health facilities—or rather a proliferation dictated
by the special needs of medical specialists or of the adventitious
availability of funds from one source or another for hospital construction or expansion.

Since market forces do not function well in the health area and
since there has been little intervention by government, what Galbraith
has termed "planning lacunae"[12] have emerged, the existence of
which is extremely important for an analysis of the efficiency of
hospitals atomistically or collectively. We must enter a basic caution
here before proceeding. Many students of the health field lapse into
what might be termed a reverse fallacy-of-composition error. It is
assumed that because the individual institution operates in a nonmarket
setting that individuals who are employed by or affiliated with the
institution are similarly "noneconomic" motivated. It might be granted
that nonpecuniary or psychic income derived from working in a
health-care setting constitutes a larger share of total income for such
workers than for others who work in profit-oriented enterprises.
That relatively large share, however, is still a minor portion of the
total as recent gains of unionism and strikes of all kinds by health
workers attest. This responsiveness to economic incentives on the
part of "human inputs" is an extremely important point to bear in
mind in evaluating any scheme for restructuring the health economy.

---

outputs being subordinate; in so-called teaching hospitals the functions
of education and research might be on a par with, or some say ahead
of patient care. This is what some writers have in mind when they
describe the hospital as a multiproduct firm.

The extent of increases in hospital costs has been illustrated above by some of the standard measures. We shall now probe somewhat more deeply into the question of the relationship between costs and efficiency with which hospital services are produced. The costs under consideration for this purpose are those incurred by the hospital and not the cost (price or charge) to the purchaser of hospital services, our assumption being that, though clearly not identical, they tend to move in the same direction and at the same rates.* The specific costs subsequently alluded to will, in any event, be either implicit in the context or otherwise made explicit.

At first blush, explanations for hospital cost inflation proferred by economists may appear contradictory. On the one hand, some economists place primary emphasis on "cost-push" as the initiating and driving force in inflation and on the other, the emphasis is on "demand pull." Seymour Harris, a long-time student of the inflationary process, stresses the former:

> In the medical area, cost-push is a vital factor in inducing inflation - more so than in the economy generally. The large rise of income of physicians and of the exploited other members of the medical team help explain the cost-push pressures in medicine. Increased cost-push pressure unless treated by anti-inflationary weapons is likely to bring inflation.[1]

---

*Corroboration for this statement is provided in Table 1.2 Chap. 1, columns 2 and 3.

Martin Feldstein one of the keenest students of health economics, stresses "demand pull":

> Increasing demand has been identified as the primary reason for the unusually rapid rate of cost increase. Rising income and more comprehensive insurance coverage (both private and public) have increased patients' willingness to pay for more and better hospital care.[2]

Are these explanations mutually exclusive or reconcilable? I hold that a synthesis of the two positions is possible, that they may be viewed as two sides of the same coin. Methodologically it is not possible to determine which came first. It is obvious, however, that once started the two factors become mutually reinforcing. If costs are rising from the input side they will generate a demand for more insurance coverage (public and private), and greater insurance coverage, as Feldstein points out, is an important ingredient of rising demand. Conversely, if increased demand is causing costs to rise the resulting increase in hospital revenues enables administrators to raise wages more easily and readily.

A digression from Feldstein's study is in order because of the importance of the inflationary mechanisms he discusses. There are a number of his points with which I take issue. First, on consumer demand, Feldstein reasons that "if hospital charges had remained constant, hospital care would have become less expensive relative to the other goods and services that consumers purchase (even if there had been no change in insurance) and the demand for care would therefore have increased."[3] This is true only if the demand for hospital care is elastic with respect to real income, that is if it is a "normal good." Most consumers would prefer to buy goods and services that yield "positive utilities" rather than goods and services that are expected to remove a negative utility, e.g. an illness; one goes to a hospital not because he expects to have a pleasant experience. A second point in Feldstein's presentation is more directly concerned with cost:

> The effect of prepaying health care through insurance, both private and government, is to encourage hospitals to produce a more expensive product than consumers actually wish to purchase. <u>At the time of illness</u>, the insured patient's demand for care reflects the <u>net</u> price, i.e. the hospital's charge net of the insurance benefits. He is therefore willing to purchase much more expensive care than he would if he were not insured.[4] [Emphasis added.]

Several demurrers must be entered here. In the first place, the consumer does not know ex ante what the net charge for his stay is going to be. Most consumers are only vaguely familiar with their insurance contracts in terms of coverage. Even if they are better informed they do not always know how long their hospital stay will be, how many and what kinds of ancillary services their physicians will order and what the charges will be for them. In short the consumer's conception of the net cost to him might be, and usually is very wide of the mark. A more fundamental objection, however, is Feldstein's apparent confusion between expensive services and inflation. In simple terms, what he has said is that—by analogy—when the consumer decides to buy a car he will buy a Buick instead of a Chevrolet. This might well be, but buying Buicks does not lead to an increase in an index of automobile prices. The confusion here is between an increase in expenditures, which do go up, with an increase in prices, which might not necessarily go up, parri passu, and may even decrease.

A word should also be said concerning Feldstein's concept of "philanthropic wage setting," which he defines as the payment of "decent" and "just" wages rather than the lowest wages at which the services can be obtained on the grounds that management in nonprofit institutions "may concern itself with the welfare of its staff as well as of its patients."[5] Perhaps one should permit Leon Davis* to speak to this point. Suffice it to say, the many strikes and near strikes of hospital employees in recent, relatively affluent times—for hospitals— casts serious doubt on the hypothesis. Moreover, the thesis is contradicted by Feldstein himself in a footnote[6] suggesting that collusion on salaries and wages might have occurred. Does it no longer take place ?

Throughout the Feldstein study little attention is paid to the general question of supply. No allowance is made for offsets to cost increases arising from internal and/or external economies. Feldstein's definition of supply increases is restricted to three components: an increase in the number of beds and personnel to staff them; an increase in the supply of nurses and other specialized personnel per bed; and an increase in capital expenditures or "modernization." Feldstein states: "Only the first of these is likely to reduce cost per patient day and all these could contribute to a higher total cost of hospital care."[7] Given Feldstein's definition of supply, he is probably correct, but increases in supply should encompass, for instance, not merely a quantitative increase in the number of beds but in the types of beds and facilities in accordance with the modern notion of

---

*Leon Davis is president of Local 1195, Drug and Hospital Workers Union.

"progressive patient care," or articulating the health structure more closely with its health function. An illustration from the recent hearings of the Senate Subcommittee on Antitrust and Monopoly may be instructive. John Freund Gillespie, an M.D. and health consultant, testified:

> In round estimates, using the $62 (as of 1968) per day
> basis, in the conventional hospital there are approximately
> 5 percent of the patients who can classify as being acutely
> ill and therefore would require an expense of approx-
> imately $100 a day. There are 15 percent classified
> subacutely ill which could be easily managed at the expense
> of approximately $60 a day. The bulk of the patients or
> 60 percent, fall into the convalescent or other chronically
> ill category and could be managed on $40 per day and the
> balance or 20 percent of the patients are ambulant or were
> admitted for diagnosis and needed only a $20 motel-like
> accommodation.[8]

A simple numerical example, assuming 100 patients, and using the ratios indicated provides these statistics:

```
            5 patients  @  100 dollars  =   500 dollars
           15 patients  @   60          =   900
           60 patients  @   40          =  2400
           20 patients  @   20          =   400
Total         100                          4200
Per patient                                  42
```

Given the actual average daily rate of $62, the new weighted average of $42 represents a saving both to the hospital and hopefully to the patient of approximately 32 percent.

With respect to Feldstein's second point—an increase in the supply of nurses, etc.—again a similar objection must be raised. It is not only a quantitative increase in personnel that is needed but a functional reallocation of personnel so that well-trained, well-paid specialists do not perform tasks for which less well-trained and well-paid employees are adequate. In a simple calculation with respect to nursing tasks suggested by the present writer several years ago, it was found that approximately $1 billion annually in nursing expenses could be saved by proper task allocation.[9] Furthermore, even after we have better matched employees to their tasks, there is still the potential of increasing productivity per worker. The combination of these two labor policies alone would unquestionably yield substantial savings in the production of hospital services since, as it is well known, payroll costs constitute roughly two/thirds of all hospital operating costs.[10]

Finally, a comment is in order on the third of Feldstein's supply components—modernization. Without going into detail, our general view is that hospitals tend to be hoarders of labor and that the substitution of capital for labor, therefore, will most probably increase productivity and, ceteris paribus, reduce unit costs. Moreover, it is plausible to assume that the physical and functional obsolescence of so large a proportion of existing hospitals results in high cost of operation.[11] While the investment of funds for modernization may in the short run result in higher cost, therefore, over a longer time horizon one might reasonably anticipate lower operating costs per unit of output, purely inflationary effects aside.

If we add to the foregoing the potential increases in productivity arising from increased hospital managerial efficiency and the potential cost reductions arising from facility mergers, from interhospital cooperation in purchasing, from centralized laboratory, food and laundry operations, and from centralized, computerized bed reservation systems, the potential for substantial and significant reduction in the cost of production of hospital services must be judged to be considerable.* Policies to accomplish these objectives must be vigorously pursued especially in view of the increase in demand that would be generated by a national health insurance system.

To return to the more analytical questions raised earlier—namely the general relationship between cost and efficiency—Feldstein makes an important distinction between technical efficiency or productivity, which has to do with the relation between the quantity of outputs produced by inputs and "economic efficiency" or "input efficiency" (some authors use the term "pecuniary efficiency"), which refers to producing a given output at least cost.[12] The first, technical efficiency, is a physical measure, the second a monetary measure. It is conceivable that there could be a divergence between the two measures. A hospital might operate with a very low ratio of payroll to total expense because it uses many volunteer workers, or, as in the case of some hospitals owned by religious orders, the workers might not be paid or might receive nominal payments. Such a hospital might be economically efficient but technically inefficient. Conversely, a hospital might be operating with an optimum combination of input factors

---

*For some examples in the United States and abroad, see, "Innovations in Hospital Management" in Hospitals, Volume 43, June 16, 1969; and "Lowering the Cost of Medical Treatment," European Public Health Committee, Council of Europe, Strasbourg, France, March 1969.

(land, capital, labor, and management) but, because of supply-demand
conditions in the market for such factors, its cost might be "high."
In fact, there is a relationship between technical and economic efficiency that is determined by the resources available to management
(the budget) and the prices of factors. In profit-seeking firms the
task of management is relatively straightforward—producing an output
at least cost. In nonprofit institutions such as voluntary hospitals
economic constraints might not be as direct as they are in business
firms, but it would be incorrect to suppose that they are non-existent.
We shall have more to say about these matters.

We have alluded to the nature of "output" in hospital production.
The output of any good or service is two-dimensional in that it has
a quantity and a quality component. In hospitals, as noted above, the
quantity component may be measured by admissions, discharges,
length of stay, patient days, outpatient visits, and other factors. The
quality component, not surprisingly, is more difficult to measure since
it too, is two-dimensional, possessing both objective and subjective
elements. As in education production, the assumption is that if inputs
are of high quality, viz., well-trained and motivated, they are likely,
all things being equal, to be reflected in the output. If a hospital
possesses highly trained and well motivated physicians and nurses,
if it has state-of-the-art equipment and a competent administration,
the quality of care received by its patients is likely to be high. In the
Appendix to Chapter 3 we utilize a surrogate for these quality factors
in attempting to measure output and productivity in the sample of
hospitals.

There is one other factor involved in the input-output relationships in hospitals that must be examined—the way in which costs
vary with the level of output. In an archetypical firm with fixed and
variable costs, the cost per unit of output will be a function of that
output. At low levels of output "overhead" or fixed costs are con-
centrated in a relatively few output units, resulting in relatively high
costs. At very high levels of output the ratio of variable to fixed costs
is similarly highly unbalanced with resulting high costs. Applying
these factors to hospital activity we would expect that the hospital's
cost-per-patient day would be high at low levels of output (say 10
percent bed occupancy or capacity) and would be high, too, at high
levels of output (say 95 percent-100 percent of capacity)* and that they
would be lower for some range of capacity between the extremes.

---

*There is sometimes a tendency to confuse maximum with optimum
output; cf. William Hickey, "Are Hospitals Using Their Capital Efficiently?" <u>Modern Hospital</u>, December 1967 and John H. Hayes,
"Factors Affecting the Costs of Hospital Care." Blakiston, 1954, p.
193 and 194.

Although most of the empirical studies of cost-output relationships in hospitals confirm the general pattern described, some
have found L-shaped and even inverted U-shaped cost curves. Until
we get more and better empirical work in this area the writer is
inclined to accept Feldstein's finding as typical that for a sample of
British hospitals:

> The average cost function, when adjusted for case-mix, is
> a shallow U-shaped curve with a minimum at the current
> average size (310 beds). Costs rise beyond this size but
> level off after 600 beds at about 10 percent above the min-
> imum cost. The failure to achieve economies of scale is
> primarily due to the lower case-bed ratio in larger hos-
> pitals, even after adjusting for case-mix differences.
> This probably reflects a lower level of "managerial" or
> labor efficiency, and, in particular, a slower hospital
> pace.[13]

Accepting the existence of a U-shaped curve we should add that
two hospitals might still vary in pecuniary efficiency even if they
are operating at the same output levels. This may be illustrated as
follows:

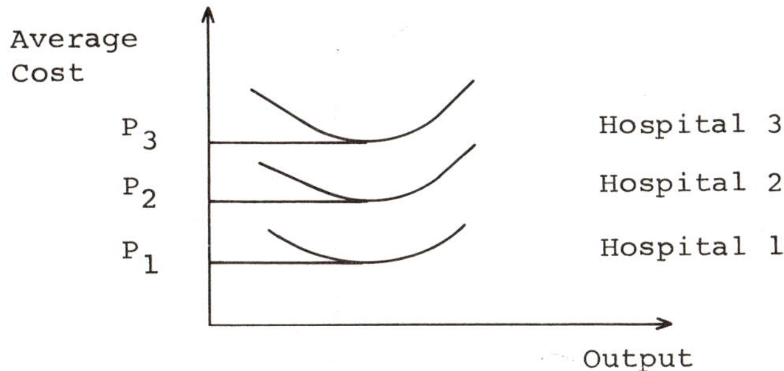

Though the cost pattern is similar, the unit cost levels of hospital 1
are lower than those of hospitals 2 and 3 over the entire output
range,[14] assuming minimum cost operation and prices at P_1, P_2,
and P_3. We shall consider the factors affecting the range of prices
from P_1 to P_3 below.
   We are now in a position to discuss some general approaches to
hospital efficiency. Whether one is interested in examining a single

hospital, a cross section of hospitals, or intertemporal comparisons, the over-all productivity of the institution may be approached by determining its total output and dividing by all or some of the inputs— labor, capital, total assets, etc. We can also disaggregate the total into departmental productivity measures—radiology, nursing, laboratory, etc.—and finally get down to individual worker productivity.

There are some policy questions that should be raised before we look at some of the details concerning efficiency. Under competitive conditions in the business sector, inefficient firms will not survive for long, as a casual look at the number of bankruptcies per year will show. In the nonprofit sector many more inefficient firms can and often do survive. To the extent that they do they serve to raise the average level of resources society devotes to health care. Should public policy therefore be aimed at eliminating inefficient hospitals? Furthermore, even if a hospital is efficient in the context of outputs and inputs, it might not be needed in a particular community for one reason or another. The implication, therefore, is that societal needs for hospitals must be balanced against the efficiency with which services are produced by individual institutions to approach some type of Pareto optimum.

THE ELUSIVE OUTPUT
AND OTHER
MEASUREMENT PROBLEMS

Our view of hospital output, again, is that it is a complex function of the number of inpatients plus outpatients treated per time period, the types of illnesses on admission, the quantity and quality of human and physical hospital resources applied to the patient, and some scalar measure of the success of treatment—zero if no effect, positive if the patient improves, and negative if the patient's condition deteriorates as a result of hospital care.

Readmissions caused by inappropriate or poor hospital treatment—iatrogenic admissions, so to speak—should be charged against the output of a hospital in much the same way that defective merchandise or merchandise returns are handled in the manufacturing and retailing sectors.

One would also wish to make adjustments to output—more specifically to the output costs—to take account of what the economist calls "neighborhood effects," or externalities. Smoke from the hospital's heating or incinerating plant, for example, raises social costs whereas the utility accruing to non-patients from the patients' treatment, such as the prevention of communicable disease, should diminish such costs. In the case of hospitals the presumption— confirmed by cost-benefit analyses—is that positive external effects far exceed the negative ones so that the net cost to society is over- stated in hospital and all health expenditure data.[1]

This chapter seeks to explore some of the conceptual and empirical problems inherent in attempts to measure output, efficiency, and costs by economists and hospital accountants to the end not of developing an "ideal" measure of efficiency but of focusing attention on a combination of factors that lie at the core of the issue.

The first and perhaps major tasks are those of focusing and clarifying issues. It is an exercise in frustration to discuss productivity measures in terms of inputs and outputs only to have someone question whether some patients needed to be hospitalized at all. As pointed out previously, many patients do not, but if they become patients in an extended care facility it is that facility or productive unit for which productivity must also be measured. Unless we simplify assumptions at the outset it will be impossible to make progress on these issues. Lest we be accused of assuming away the problems, we assume explicitly—and these assumptions will be relaxed—that the patients require hospitalization, that they are treated in a state-of-the-medical-art fashion both in terms of trained manpower and facilities, and that there are no extraneous factors such as insurance contracts that induce manipulation of the length of their stay. Given these assumptions we can measure the efficiency with which hospital services are produced both in physical, or engineering terms and in value, or monetary terms. The efficiency measure so calculated will then be a function of managerial expertise and employee skills and motivation, as well as of the age of the hospital plant, its design, its degree of utilization, and the state of its equipment.

It has always amazed me to see critiques of hospital rates couched in terms of the dispersion of per diem costs or hospital rates in a given area.[2] With all of the factors just cited, whereby hospitals of even the same approximate size and type might differ, rate variation is to be expected and rate uniformity would have to be ascribed to coincidence, to collusion, or to external regulation.

Our simplified assumptions also permit an easy solution to a problem that has perplexed many researchers, namely the question of the choice of the output unit. For instance, if two patients occupy two beds, and remain in the hospital for 100 days, the output of the hospital may be said to be 200 bed or patient days. That same output would result if 100 patients occupied beds for two days apiece. Clearly, any measure that disregarded the way in which the total 200 patient day output was generated would conceal more than it revealed, even though it were technically correct. If our assumption that patients are provided state-of-the-art services is granted, however, we may postulate further an average length of stay per patient—say, of eight days. It would then be a matter of indifference whether total patient days or total cases treated (the quotient of bed days and the average length of stay) was used as the output measure. In practice the American Hospital Association (AHA) and other sources of hospital data use the patient day measure thus presenting analysts with the very problem just discussed.

There remains a serious ambiguity with respect to the patient day output measure that must be dealt with at this point. Feldstein, commenting on a paper of Melvin Reder's, has formulated it clearly:

> The dividing line between inputs and outputs is unclear.
> For me, the distinguishing characteristic is the possi-
> bility of substitution. Although Reder classifies a hospital
> bed day as an input, I would treat it as a form of output
> because it can be produced with different combinations
> of inputs. I would not deny, of course, that a bed day is
> also an input used in producing the output, "a treated
> case." But a treated case is also an input in producing
> an improvement in the community's health level.[3]

I believe that Feldstein is correct, but not for the reasons he gives. After all, it is sometimes possible to substitute ambulatory care for inpatient care, as implied in his statement, so the input combination criterion can be used in support of both positions. Nor does it prevent one from specifying something as an output that is used again as an input. The output of a bolt shop is a bolt, even though it might be used in the construction of a car. Whether we specify an output as intermediate or as final depends on the problem at hand. If the problem is one of determining the efficiency of a hospital, then patient days, appropriately adjusted, constitute the proper output.

Herbert Klarman has raised another problem with respect to the use of patient days as an output measure:

> The assumption that the hospital patient day represents a
> constant unit of service is contradicted by experience. It
> is possible to devise a measure of the change in activity
> in hospitals by recognizing that the volume of ancillary
> services rendered in the hospital (such as laboratory or
> radiology) may be more closely associated with the num-
> ber of admissions than with the number of patient days.[4]

As we have pointed out, it is possible to use a variety of meas-ures, of which admissions is one, to determine the level of activity or the rate of resource utilization in hospitals. Each measure has its advantages and disadvantages. The problem thus becomes one either of using several indicators simultaneously or of settling on one measure that comes closest to approximating the aggregate activity level. The weakness of the admissions measure is similar to our earlier demonstration with respect to patient days and may be illus-trated as follows: Assume 100 admissions to a hospital. Two of the patients admitted are discharged after spending one day in the hospital; the other 98 remain in the hospital for 50 days. Clearly, using the admissions measure alone would not provide an indicator of the amount and types of resources used to treat those admitted. It might be objected that Klarman opted not for admissions as a measure but for

ancillary activities associated with admissions. Again, there is nothing
inherently incorrect in using such measures as the number of laboratory
tests per annum, the number of x-rays per annum, the number of meals
served, the pounds of laundry processed, or total payroll as output
measures, but they are all partial rather than aggregate indexes and,
used separately, fall short of an over-all measure of hospital productivity. They are similarly unsatisfactory measures of the specific
"value added" contribution of hospitals to total output.

When we move from quantitative to qualitative output considerations the road becomes even more slippery. In evaluating medical
school quality we can point to the Flexner Report of 1910 as marking
the beginning of the transition from "diploma mills" to the high quality,
academically and scientifically oriented medical schools of today.
This is not to imply that all medical schools are of uniformly high
quality, rather that the dispersion of quality institutions is much less
now than it was before Flexner called attention to the problem. The
hospital field <u>per se</u> has not had its "Flexner Report," although one
can point to a long series of official and semiofficial reports on the
nation's hospitals beginning with the deliberations of the Committee
on the Costs of Medical Care in the early 1930s. Improvements in
the nation's hospitals have thus been slower than they have been in
medical schools; the Joint Commission on Accreditation of Hospitals,
for example, was not founded until 1952. The Somers' Report of 1965
indicated that "some 62 percent of short-term hospitals with 87 percent
of the beds listed by AHA, were accredited."[5] Four years later, these
ratios were 71 and 91 respectively.* Undoubtedly the evolution of
hospital quality improvement received a great fillip from the Medicare
and Medicaid amendments to the Social Security Act of 1965, which
required that hospitals meet certain minimal standards if they were
to participate, i.e. be reimbursed for care in these programs.

Although over-all quality has improved, quality differences
among hospitals persist. The major factors accounting for such
differences are hospital size and type, medical school affiliation,
location, number of facilities and services, degree of modernization,
and the amount and types of medical specialists on the staff. In this
chapter we shall utilize the number of services available as a proxy
for general quality.

Quality differences cause at least two important measurement
problems: A patient day of care in a 25-bed hospital does not have
the same resource content as one in a 1,000-bed hospital. A patient
day of care in 1970 might not have had the same resource content as
one in 1965, even in the same hospital. Point one I think, will be

---

*<u>Guide Issue</u>, August 1, 1970, p. 456.

readily conceded, but what are the differences, if any, between a 400 and a 450-bed hospital? In point two, a computation by Feldstein is apposite. He indicates that, "hospitals used some 63 percent more real resources [labor and nonlabor inputs] per patient day in 1968 than they had thirteen years earlier, an average annual increase of 3.8 percent."[6] On the assumption that the increased resources used are not a result of decreasing productivity, and that they bear some relationship to the level of care, it is likely that the quality of a patient day care is now higher than in previous periods.

Feldstein derives some extremely important conclusions from these facts:

> . . . [A] day of hospital care is a product that has been continually changing. The rising cost of hospital care is therefore not comparable to price increases for other goods and services that consumers buy. Moreover, the changing character of the product implies that cost increases should not be interpreted as evidence of inefficiency or a low rate of technical progress.[7]

The crucial question, of course, is whether cost increases exceed those mandated by necessary increases in wage costs and by the incorporation of technological (informational and instrumental) advances into the hospital. The evidence we have seen,[8] some of which will be evaluated below, supports the presumption that a not inconsiderable portion of the increase arises from such factors as the monopolistic position of hospital-based specialists such as pathologists, radiologists, and anesthesiologists, or internal resources misallocation, a non-rationalized production scheduling system, a dysfunctional reimbursement system, or a diffuse intrahospital and interhospital control system, to cite some of the more important factors.

More generally, we hold with Leibenstein that at any given time "sub-optimal disequilibrium with respect to technology and utilization of existing capital stock is prevalent and important—apart from new capital infusions or changes in technique."[9] If this is true of profit-seeking firms, it applies _a fortiori_ to those, like voluntary hospitals, in the nonprofit sector.

We turn now from more abstract measurement concepts to pragmatic problems of measurement faced by those in charge of the accounting of hospital activities. Our main purpose here is to determine the extent to which the measurement of hospital accounts might be used as a managerial tool for promoting efficiency.

I should like at the outset to cite a general bias of economists with respect to accounting practice, namely that the valuation of capital assets as well as annual depreciation charges against those assets should be based on replacement cost, i.e., current value rather than historical cost, i.e., value at time of purchase. I am aware that this entails the calculation of price indexes and the periodic adjustment of original costs, but these are not inherently complex. The all too common alternative—that of using historical cost—seriously understates the rate of capital resource use and therefore is not a useful guide to capital investment decisions. Moreover, as one authority in hospital accounting put it: "The fact that a rapidly rising price level, in combination with historical cost basis of depreciation, produces losses even where accounting "profits" are reported, is not generally understood."[10]

Apart from problems of internal resource allocation, accounting techniques are the means whereby costs and charges are determined and through these the links among hospitals, patients, and third-party payers are forged.

A systematic study of hospital accounting practices was made feasible by two AHA publications—"Chart of Accounts for Hospitals" (1966) and "Cost Finding and Rate Setting for Hospitals" (1968). Prior to these publications, and in keeping with the prevailing autonomous and uncoordinated hospital (government hospitals excepted) system, each facility used its own accounting techniques and definitions so that one could not determine the financial position of even a single hospital with confidence, much less make comparisons among hospitals in terms of standard accounting ratios and criteria. While complete uniformity has by no means been achieved, continuous exhortations and flow of educational materials by the AHA, Blue Cross, State Health departments, and now the Social Security Administration under Title 18 and Title 19 have brought about marked improvements in the quality of hospital reporting.

While improved statistical and financial measurement within hospitals is desirable in itself, there are important objectives that it should serve. The governing authority or administration should utilize reporting techniques as tools to promote internal efficiency, attempt to minimize cost operation for a given output level, and assure the orderly growth of the institution consonant with community needs and desires. The prevention of deleterious practices should also be high on management's agenda. An example of the latter problem is the proclivity toward departmental empire building, which, because of the power of the technostructure (see chapter 1), appears to be endemic to hospital organization. L. Vann Seawell has pointed out: "In order to restrain such tendencies, hospital management must have the ability to recognize overinvestment and inefficient use of capital within departments of the hospital."[11] And while it is easier said than done, L. Vann Seawell urges continuous flexibility with respect to the kinds of data the decision makers receive, for, he notes, "reports, once established in a hospital, soon take on an aura of tradition and are continued just because they have been used in the past."[12]

C. Rufus Rorem, one of the most creative thinkers in the field of hospital management, was, in my view, most conservative when he stated: "There is convincing evidence that more careful attention to accounting records and reports and the application of these data to hospital management could achieve at least a five percent increase in hospital service without additional expenditure."[13]

Finally, mention should be made of what, in economic theory at least, are the two basic functions of management—to earn profits (the time period is sticky here) and to minimize losses (thus maintaining the firm as a going concern). In nonprofit hospitals, as we have observed, the first function is, by definition, not applicable. What of the second? Accountants are likely to be particularistic at this point, as Vann Seawall illustrates:

> A hospital which incurs operating losses over a period of
> years, or just manages to break even, may actually render
> a disservice to the community it serves. A hospital with
> continual and substantial operating losses will be unable
> to maintain capable personnel and keep up to date in life-
> saving equipment.[14]

I can think of no more effective counterview to this argument than a statement by John H. Hayes made ten years before the publication of the Vann Seawell book:

> The studies of the Commission [on Financing of Hospital
> Care] indicate that a deficit in a particular year does not
> necessarily indicate either poor management or lack of
> community support. More often a deficit reflects the
> instability of hospital financing, which makes precise
> planning difficult. Typically, hospitals attempt to limit
> operating expense to an amount equal to the anticipated
> income from all sources. Success or failure in balancing
> income and expense is not in itself an indication of success
> or failure in meeting community needs. A hospital should
> neither fear a deficit nor be proud of its existence. To
> carry out needed expansion of a service program may
> require the courage to risk the occurrence of a deficit.[15]

If one were to include social or community welfare in the accounting system, it is quite possible that a hospital with deficits might, in fact, be of greater value than one with consistent surpluses. The fact is, however, that while nominally called "community hospitals,"

the voluntaries are autonomous entities issuing their own annual
reports and functioning with their own internal or, for the most part,
external constituencies. It might well be that achieving some admixture
of the Vann Seawell and Hayes approaches reflects the central problem
of the contemporary hospital economy.

APPENDIX

An Approach to the Measurement of
Hospital Output and Productivity

In developing the analogy of the hospital as a firm we soon
arrive at the point of measuring total output as well as productivity—
output per unit of input. In general calculation of these measures
increases in complexity as we proceed from simple goods production
and becomes even more complex when we are dealing with the output
of services. Within the services sector the subgroups education and
health pose the most formidable conceptual problems.

At several points we have indicated our general agreement with
specification of the patient day as an appropriate output measure for
hospitals. It will be recalled, however, that the support for this
measure was conditional on making "appropriate adjustments."

The first and most obvious of these adjustments concerns the
necessity of combining what heretofore have been treated as uncom-
binable outputs, namely inpatient days of care and outpatient care.
The main components of the latter are visits to outpatient and
emergency rooms. Strangely enough, it was not until 1969 that the
AHA in its annual Guide Issue of Hospitals, for the first time in its
25 years of publication, combined inpatient and outpatient care in its
statistical section:

> In recognition [sic] of the need for a single measure of
> hospital services, a new measure, incorporating both
> inpatient and outpatient care services, has been developed.
> In the simplest terms, this new measure converts the num-
> ber of outpatient visits into units roughly equivalent to an
> inpatient day in level of effort in economic terms, reflect-
> ing utilization of both manpower and facilities. The com-
> bination of these equivalent patient days and the actual
> inpatient days produces a new measure called adjusted
> patient days.[16]

It is not clear, and the subsequent discussion in the Guide Issue
makes it dubious, whether emergency room visits are considered as
a part of outpatient visits. If they are not, it would be a serious

omission since 90 percent of community hospitals report operating
emergency departments, and such visits have been rising rapidly,
especially in inner-city facilities.[17]

The method employed by the AHA to effect the combination of
inpatient and outpatient visits was to divide inpatient revenue per
patient day by outpatient revenue per outpatient visit to produce a
"corrective factor, indicating the number of outpatient visits necessary
to equal one day of inpatient care in terms of level of effort."[18]

Unfortunately it is not "level of effort" but pricing policies that
are reflected by this technique. Unless all prices for services are set
equal to the costs of producing those services, or unless the two are
systematically related—for example, if prices were set at "X" percent
above costs—revenues do not necessarily reflect resource use. This
is especially true when hospitals are reimbursed for services rendered
on a "reasonable cost" or even on a "cost-plus" basis. While the
AHA should be commended for attempting, at long last, a solution to
the total output problem, it would appear that with refined accounting
techniques available multiple cost-finding for inpatient, outpatient,
and emergency room services should be more directly calculable so
that the correction factor would more nearly approach effort levels.

The AHA technique yielded an average correction factor of 4.9
for 1968, 4.9 outpatient visits being equivalent to one inpatient day of
care, that factor generally varying inversely with hospital bed size.
In the calculations that follow, and in accordance with data provided
by the Associated Hospital Service of New York (Blue Cross),[19] we
use three outpatient visits and four emergency room visits as the
equivalent of one day of inpatient care for New York hospitals
irrespective of size.

The second major problem with respect to the measure of output
is the quality factor. Irving Leveson has stated this problem suc-
cinctly:

> The standard economic models deal with a simple homo-
> geneous product. Inefficiency occurs simply as high unit
> costs. Where quality can vary widely, as in the production
> of many publicly funded services, it becomes important
> to analyze efficiency in terms of quality as well.[20]

There is a large and growing body of literature on the question
of medical quality that is beyond the scope of this study to evaluate.
We take it that there is an overwhelming consensus on the view that
generally, if not invariably, the quality of medical care rendered by
large hospitals is superior to, or on a higher level than that rendered
by small hospitals. For instance, whereas only 15 percent of the
hospitals in the under-25-bed category reported postoperative
recovery room services, 100 percent of the 500-and-over-bed hospitals

TABLE 3.1

Quality Adjusted Patient Day Calculations for
Selected Hospitals, 400 Beds and Over

Year	Hospital	Number of Beds	Number of Employees	Number of Services	Quality Proxy	Inpatient Days	Outpatient Visits
1970	Presbyterian Hospital	1,568	5,017	28	.85	447,004	391,824
1969	Society of the New York Hospital	1,510	4,359	28	.85	434,061	245,023
1969	Mount Sinai Hospital	1,176	3,327	31	.94	410,808	492,018
1969	Montefiore Hospital	1,168	5,664	31	.94	403,234	152,547
1969	St. Vincent's Hospital and Medical Center	953	2,864	33	100	276,600	71,523
1968	Kingsbrook Jewish Medical Center	822	1,548	24	.73	275,621	22,016
1969	St. Luke's Hospital Center	713	3,116	26	.79	223,745	165,284
1969	Jewish Hospital and Medical Center of Brooklyn	602	2,110	24	.73	217,211	63,847
1970	Roosevelt Hospital	595	2,757	29	.88	201,549	163,448
1968	Long Island College Hospital	575	1,743	27	.82	188,164	49,305
1969	Maimonides Medical Center	565	2,126	29	.88	169,623	52,123
1969	Bronx Lebanon Medical Center	564	1,864	22	.67	189,351	129,984
1969	Methodist Hospital of Brooklyn	469	1,293	26	.79	205,860	37,000
1970	Long Is. Jewish Medical Center	450	1,800	25	.76	135,000	36,000
1969	St. Clare's Hospital	410	1,204	24	.73	128,119	25,720
	Local Government Institutions						
1969	Nassau County Medical Center	631	1,845	28	.82	169,509	123,146
1969	Kings County Hospital Center	2,272	5,325	34	1.00	666,490	439,006
1969	Harlem Hospital Center	910	3,900	27	.79	269,293	23,308

Year	Hospital	Outpatient Equivalent (6) ÷ 3	Emergency Room Visits	Emergency Visit Equivalent (8) ÷ 4	Adjusted Patient Days (5) + (7) + (9)	Quality Adjusted Patient Days (10) x (4)	QAPD per Employee (11) ÷ (2)
1970	Presbyterian Hospital	130,614	37,022	9,256	586,874	497,953	99
1969	Society of the New York Hospital	81,674	34,291	8,573	524,808	444,867	102
1969	Mount Sinai Hospital	164,006	96,360	24,158	568,972	534,488	161
1969	Montifiore Hospital	50,849	37,643	9,410	463,493	435,683	70
1969	St. Vincent's Hospital and Medical Center	23,841	48,193	12,048	312,489	312,489	109
1968	Kingsbrook Jewish Medical Center	7,339	2,330	583	283,542	206,212	133
1969	St. Luke's Hospital Center	55,095	87,206	21,802	300,641	236,869	76
1969	Jewish Hospital and Medical Center of Brooklyn	21,282	45,813	11,453	249,949	181,781	86
1970	Roosevelt Hospital	54,483	61,302	15,326	271,357	238,465	86
1968	Long Island College Hospital	16,433	30,190	7,548	212,147	173,574	100
1969	Maimonides Medical Center	17,374	41,427	10,357	197,354	173,432	82
1969	Bronx Lebanon Medical Center	43,328	59,290	14,823	247,502	161,005	86
1969	Methodist Hospital of Brooklyn	12,333	41,000	10,250	228,443	179,986	139
1970	Long Island Jewish Medical Center	12,000	30,000	7,500	154,500	117,045	65
1969	St. Clare's Hospital	8,573	20,419	5,105	141,797	103,125	86
	Local Government Institutions						
1969	Nassau County Medical Center	41,048	58,836	14,709	225,266	185,511	100
1969	Kings County Hospital Center	146,335	188,227	47,057	859,882	859,882	162
1969	Harlem Hospital Center	77,693	122,705	30,676	377,662	299,905	77

Source: Annual Reports; Guide Issue - 1969 and 1970; Health and Hospital Planning Council of Southern New York

TABLE 3.2

Quality Adjusted Patient Day Calculations For
Selected Hospitals, 200 - 400 Beds

		Number of Beds	Number of Employees	Number of Services	Quality Proxy	In-Patient Days	Out-Patient Visits	Out-Patient Equivalent (6) ÷ 3 = (7)
1969	Mercy Hospital	386	1057	25	.93	131,638	13,019	4,440
1969	United Hospital	365	828	22	.82	104,755	—	—
1968	Polyclinic Hospital	333	796	17	.63	103,444	37,031	12,344
1969	Misericordia Hospital	332	1175	25	.93	110,432	120,159	40,053
1970	Hospital for Joint Diseases	330	862	22	.82	106,278	62,485	20,828
1969	Flushing Hospital and Medical Center	326	825	23	.85	109,485	11,238	3,746
1968	South Nassau Communities Hospital	321	854	22	.82	100,361	—	—
1969	Vassar Brothers Hospital	310	698	22	.82	98,550	—	—
1969	St. Vincent's Medical Center of Richmond	310	984	19	.70	105,554	25,631	8,544
1970	North Shore Hospital	307	965	26	.96	116,133	31,220	10,407
1969	Lawrence Hospital	300	623	19	.70	87,221	2,356	785
1969	Huntington Hospital	295	814	16	.59	104,901	—	—
1966	Columbus Hospital	288	681	20	.74	97,490	17,450	5,817
1969	Lutheran Hospital Center	288	848	19	.70	105,249	46,685	15,562
1969	Benedictine Hospital	280	437	11	.41	71,961	—	—
1969	Jamaica Hospital	276	817	19	.70	88,995	19,684	6,561
1969	Staten Island Hospital	276	722	18	.67	93,222	17,950	5,983
1967	New York Infirmary	265	757	18	.67	79,088	26,464	8,821
1969	White Plains Hospital	262	650	19	.70	74,065	—	—
1969	Elizabeth A. Horton Hospital	256	573	23	.85	84,385	—	—
1969	St. Luke's Hospital	251	570	16	.59	83,347	—	—
1969	Booth Memorial Hospital	250	794	19	.70	98,066	12,297	4,099
1969	Southside Hospital	248	548	20	.74	79,059	—	—
1968	French Hospital	238	601	17	.63	74,385	18,599	6,200
1968	St. Joseph's Hospital	223	735	11	.41	75,727	7,840	2,613
1968	New York Eye and Ear Infirmary	207	533	9	.33	51,400	95,789	31,930
1969	Hospital for Special Surgery	204	744	10	.37	61,095	34,394	11,465
1969	Beekman Downtown Hospital	200	437	19	.70	71,961	—	—

		Emergency Room Visits	Emergency Visit Equivalent (8) ÷ (4)	Adjusted Patient Days (5) + (7) + (9)	Q.A.P.D. (10) x (4)	Q.A.P.D. per Employee (11) − (2)
1969	Mercy Hospital	14,493	3,623	139,601	129,259	122
1969	United Hospital	—	—	104,753	85,355	103
1968	Polyclinic Hospital	20,668	5,167	120,954	76,156	96
1969	Misericordia Hospital	73,834	18,456	168,944	156,428	133
1970	Hospital for Joint Diseases	21,537	5,384	132,491	107,955	125
1969	Flushing Hospital and Medical Center	22,085	5,521	118,752	101,159	123
1968	South Nassau Communities Hospital	13,625	3,406	103,767	86,995	102
1969	Vassar Brothers Hospital	—	—	98,550	80,300	115
1969	St. Vincent's Medical Center of Richmond	25,478	6,370	120,467	84,773	86
1970	North Shore Hospital	—	—	126,540	121,853	126
1969	Lawrence Hospital	10,077	2,519	90,526	63,703	102
1969	Huntington Hospital	25,068	6,267	111,168	65,877	81
1966	Columbus Hospital	9,473	2,368	105,675	78,278	115
1969	Lutheran Hospital	39,527	9,882	130,693	91,968	109
1969	Benedictine Hospital	—	—	71,961	29,317	67
1969	Jamaica Hospital	36,091	9,023	104,579	73,592	90
1969	Staten Island Hospital	18,636	4,659	103,774	69,182	96
1967	New York Infirmary	—	—	87,909	58,606	77
1969	White Plains Hospital	19,405	4,851	78,916	55,533	85
1969	Elizabeth A. Horton Hospital	10,680	2,670	87,055	74,158	129
1969	St. Luke's Hospital	27,842	6,961	90,307	53,515	94
1969	Booth Memorial Hospital	1,770	4,426	106,591	75,008	95
1969	Southside Hospital	36,874	9,219	88,276	65,391	119
1968	French Hospital	13,101	3,575	84,160	52,989	88
1968	St. Joseph's Hospital	16,584	4,146	82,486	33,605	46
1968	New York Eye and Ear Infirmary	5,963	1,491	84,821	28,273	53
1969	Hospital for Special Surgery	—	—	72,560	26,874	36
1969	Beekman Downtown Hospital	—	—	66,065	46,490	89

<u>Source</u>: Same as Table 3.1.

offered such services. Again, whereas only five percent of the under-
25-bed facilities offered intensive care units, 99 percent of the larger
ones did, and so on.[21] These are objective correlates of quality
that, in my view, are preferable to subjective evaluations of quality
care actually received by patients. Consumers of health care lack
the requisite knowledge by which to judge medical quality; what is
usually mistaken for high quality is in fact "bedside manner." I do
not wish to diminish the importance of kind words in the alleviation
of anxiety. When a patient is deeply anesthetized, however, he can't
hear these words; even if he could they would be poor substitutes for
skillful surgical knowledge and performance, complex monitoring
equipment, and the availability of the services noted above.

There are four readily available objective indexes of hospital
quality: The Directory of Approved Internships and Residencies,
a measure of how professional organizations view the facilities and
personnel of a given hospital; The National Intern and Resident
Matching Program, a measure of how medical school graduates
view the same factors; the number of approvals received by a
hospital, which partly overlaps with the first index but also includes
assessment by government authorities who must approve institutions
for participation in Medicare; and the actual facilities and services
"available within and reported by the institution."* Undoubtedly there
is a high degree of correlation among all four indexes and also between
these indexes and the size of a hospital, as even a casual perusal of
the Guide Issue of Hospitals will reveal. In one sense, the fourth
index precedes the others because a hospital does not normally
receive approvals unless its facilities have been inspected. It is for
this reason that we use the number of facilities as the quality proxy
in our calculations.

There are two (and probably more) obvious deficiencies in this
quality measure. First, it treats all services equally, i.e., unweighted
by resource use, etc. Second, it ignores quality differences within
services. The intensive care unit of one hospital, for example,
might itself be of a higher quality than that of another.† Our view,
quite simply, is that the potential benefits to be derived from using the
quality proxy outweigh the negative effects of not using such a measure
at all. Hopefully the measure will be refined by other investigators.

---

*A list of the latter is included as Exhibit A in this appendix.
†A further assumption inherent in this approach is that there
is a high, though not necessarily perfect correlation between our
quality proxy and the average annual mix of patients, "case-load
mix," thus obviating the need to deal with the latter as an independent
factor.

The objective of this study is to present a first approximation only to the measure of hospital output and productivity.

The two major adjustments for total output and for quality have been explained. Two other operating principles remain to be noted before we analyze computations. The first concerns our method of treating data and flows in part from our view of hospital size. It is manifestly unfair and substantively almost barren to compare a 1,000-bed medical school affiliated teaching hospital with a 50-bed hospital. We have therefore divided our sample of hospitals into three categories: small hospitals—those with less than 200 beds; medium sized hospitals—those with beds in the 200 to 400 range; and large hospitals—those with over 400 beds. These divisions are somewhat arbitrary and many studies utilize a greater number of subgroups but, given the number of hospitals whose annual reports we studied, this was the most expedient grouping. The second operating procedure, which also stems from our view of the importance of the size variable, concerns our treatment of the quality proxy noted earlier. For the same reasons that 50- and 1,000-bed hospitals are not comparable, the facilities and services offered are incomparable, with a few exceptions. Our method of dealing with this problem was to determine the hospital with the most facilities within each of the three groups and to set that number equal to 100. The quality proxy assigned to each of the other hospitals in its peer group was then the ratio of the number of its services divided by the highest number in the group. These ratios were used as quality weights, that is multiplied by the adjusted output (total patient days) to produce what we have termed a "quality adjusted patient day," our output measure. Restated simply, the calculation is as follows:

[Total Inpatient Days + 1/3 Outpatient Visits +
1/4 Emergency Room Visits] x Quality Proxy = Total
Quality Adjusted Patient Days (QAPD)]

The sample of hospitals we worked with was taken from the southern New York region including New York City as well as surrounding urban and suburban areas. Although it was our original intention to use data from all types of hospitals, a lack of comparable statistics restricted us to a consideration primarily of voluntary hospitals and several municipal institutions.

Results

Table 3.1 provides data on private voluntary hospitals in the larger size class—hospitals with over 400 beds. The final three

TABLE 3.3

Quality Adjusted Patient Day Calculations For
Selected Hospitals, Under 200 Beds

		Number of Beds	Number of Employees	Number of Services	Quality Proxy	In-Patient Days	Out-Patient Visits
1969	Peninsula General Hospital	195	650	22	100	63607	9483
1969	Nyack Hospital	188	528	18	.82	64866	36197
1969	Yonkers General Hospital	188	423	18	.82	60720	2949
1969	Good Samaritan Hospital	187	511	15	.68	64864	—
1969	Manhattan Eye, Ear and Throat Hospital	176	454	11	.50	47120	26220
1969	La Guardia Hospital	169	434	13	.59	62663	—
1969	St. Charles Hospital	168	549	22	100	60060	24170
1969	Southampton Hospital	146	342	15	.68	41618	—
1969	Eastern Long Island Hospital	68	142	8	.36	18994	—
1969	Midtown Hospital	60	111	7	.32	16174	—

	Out-Patient Equivalent (6) ÷ 3	Emergency Room Visits	Emergency Visit Equivalent (8) ÷ 4	Adjusted Patient Days (5) + (7) + (9)	Q.A.P.D. (10) x (4) - 100	Q.A.P.D. per Employee (11) ÷ (2)
1969 Peninsula General Hospital	3161	16553	4138	70906	70906	109
1969 Nyack Hospital	12066	18787	4697	81629	66787	126
1969 Yonkers General Hospital	983	13367	3342	65045	53218	126
1969 Good Samaritan Hospital	—	27006	6752	71616	48828	96
1969 Manhattan Eye, Ear and Throat Hospital	8740	—	—	55860	27930	62
1969 La Guardia Hospital	—	7726	1932	64594	38169	88
1969 St. Charles Hospital	8057	9299	2325	70442	70442	128
1969 Southampton Hospital	—	10379	2595	44213	30145	88
1969 Eastern Long Island Hospital	—	1647	412	19406	7057	50
1969 Midtown Hospital	—	1138	285	16459	5237	47

Source: Same as Table 3.1.

TABLE 3.4

Changes in Quality Adjusted Patient Day Per Employee For
Selected Hospitals, 1960-69

	1960 QAPD Per Employee	1970 QAPD Per Employee	Percent Change 1960-70
400 Beds and Over			
Presbyterian Hospital	178	99	-45
Society of the New York Hospital	141	102	-28
Mount Sinai Hospital	166	161	-3
Montefiore Hospital	115	70	-44
St. Vincent's Hospital and Medical Center	179	109	-39
St. Luke's Hospital Center	130	76	-41
Jewish Hospital and Medical Center, Brooklyn	140	86	-38
Roosevelt Hospital	118	86	-27
Long Island College Hospital	178	100	-44
Maimondes Medical Center	162	82	-49
Bronx Lebanon Hospital Center	136	86	-37
St. Barnabas Hospital for Chronic Diseases	222	97	-56
Memorial Hospital for Cancer	57	44	-22
Methodist Hospital of Brooklyn	99	139	+41
Long Island Jewish Medical Center	121	65	-46
St. Clare's Hospital	133	86	-35
200-400 Beds			
Hospital for Joint Diseases	186	125	-33
Flushing Hospital and Medical Center	126	123	-3
St. Vincent's Medical Center of Richmond	157	86	-45
Jamaica Hospital	114	90	-21
Staten Island Hospital	104	96	-8
New York Infirmary	122	77	-37
French Hospital	142	88	-38
St. Joseph's Hospital	87	46	-47
New York Eye and Ear Infirmary	155	53	-66
Hospital for Special Surgery	124	36	-71
Beekman Downtown Hospital	129	89	-31
Less than 200 Beds			
Manhattan Eye, Ear and Throat	114	61	-46
St. Charles Hospital	97	128	+30

Source: Same as Table 3.1.

columns are of major interest for our purposes. With respect to the differences between inpatient and quality adjusted patient days it might be noted that in more than half of the cases adjusted days were fewer than unadjusted. In other words, adjusting for non-inpatient service and for "quality" resulted in a change in the rank order by output. The final column, output per employee, also shows a change from the unadjusted output employee ratio. But the absolute figures are also of interest. Adjusted patient days per employee ranged from a high of 160 to a low of 44 with a mean for this group of 96. Interestingly, the mean adjusted output per employee of the large governmental institutions Table 3.1 was higher—133; our sample, however, was much smaller.

It is highly probable that this output per employee measure is understated because included in the employee total are those whose work is associated with the educational and research arms of the hospital and who as a consequence are functionally, in many cases even physically remote from patient day generating activities. Greater refinement of this measure, therefore, would be achieved by deducting from the denominator an amount that determined on a case-by-case basis represents the "non-patient day productive employees."

Tables 3.2 and 3.3 present similar data for the medium and smaller hospitals. A most interesting result is the practically identical average output per employee in the 200-400 bed range compared with the larger hospitals. The average of the smaller hospitals was lower—92—but this represented a differential of only four percent.

Perhaps one of the most significant uses of these calculations is the comparison of productivity over time. Table 3.4 shows changes in QAPD (Quality Adjusted Patient Day) per employee between 1960 and 1969. Of the 29 hospitals of all sizes for which we could calculate like ratios, 27 showed a decrease in output per employee over the period. This result conforms generally with the findings of the AHA, namely that "the number of community hospital employees per 1,000 adjusted patient days increased from 6.0 to 6.8 over the six year period from 1963 to 1968 or by 13 percent,"[22] although our calculations result in much larger productivity decreases. Several caveats however, should be entered before one draws conclusions regarding employee productivity. Although we use total employees in the denominator, it cannot be inferred that they are the sole input factor since capital and management are also responsible for the numerator (the output). Obviously more refined and disaggregated measures are required to separate out productivity by individual factor inputs. Nevertheless, the general decline in productivity pointed to by our aggregate measure is the real or physical base that accounts in part for the rising money costs of hospital services.

EXHIBIT A

Facilities and Services Actually available within,
and reported by, the institution

1. Intensive care unit
2. Intensive cardiac care unit
3. Open-heart surgery facilities
4. Postoperative recovery room
5. Premature nursery
6. X-ray therapy
7. Cobalt therapy
8. Radium therapy
9. Radioisotope facility
10. Histopathology laboratory
11. Organ bank
12. Blood bank
13. Electroencephalography
14. Physical therapy department
15. Occupational therapy department
16. Inhalation therapy department
17. Full-time registered pharmacist
18. Part-time registered pharmacist
19. Dental services
20. Renal dialysis, inpatient
21. Renal dialysis, outpatient
22. Self-care unit
23. Emergency department
24. Psychiatric inpatient unit
25. Psychiatric outpatient unit
26. Psychiatric partial hospitalization program
27. Psychiatric emergency services
28. Social work department
29. Family planning service
30. Extended care unit
31. Rehabilitation services, inpatient unit
32. Rehabilitation services, outpatient unit
33. Home care program
34. Hospital auxiliary
35. Organized outpatient department

Source: Hospitals, Guide Issue, August 1, 1970 pp 10-11.

Second, our method of taking quality into account, while it might enable us to say something about the relative status of a hospital within a group, cannot tell us what happens to a single institution over time. That is to say, even if hospital "A" offered the same number of facilities and services in 1960 that it did in 1969, we do not know in the absence of supplementary measures whether the quality of the same services remained constant, improved, or decreased. Third, these findings of aggregate productivity decrease are not inconsistent with what I would term a productivity increase per case or per disease. To the extent that average length of stay or length of stay per diagnostic category has decreased, one may speak of productivity as having increased. For the institution as a whole, however, operating 365 days a year and providing inpatient as well as outpatient services, the evidence points to increased unit labor or total costs even when adjusted for quality changes and decreasing length of stay.

With all their deficiencies, it is hoped that the measures proposed here will prove useful enough so that other researchers might be led to refine and extend them.[23] In undertaking this task, I have been guided by a remark of Zvi Griliches to the effect that just because it is difficult to measure something is no reason not to make a start.[24]

Considerable interhospital variation in total output per employee
and quality were revealed by the data and calculations in the previous
chapter. Two problems of economic policy are posed by these
variations: how to bring low-productivity hospitals to higher levels
and how to reduce unit costs of output even of high-productivity
hospitals, holding quality constant or, if possible, improving it.
Accordingly the present chapter focuses on intrahospital measures
for achieving operational and pecuniary efficiency. The succeeding
chapter deals with these problems from an interhospital viewpoint.

Just as Keynes alerted us to the possibility of the existence of
underemployment equilibrium, Leibenstein has alerted us to the
existence of "nonminimal cost equilibrium,"[1] that is to say that
firms may—and do—operate at output levels far from minimum cost
regions, and even if they are operating at the low point of the
average cost curve, the curve itself has the potential for downward
shifts.* In the profit sector, competitive forces might induce firms
to move from nonminimal cost positions, but in an industry that is
predominantly nonprofit oriented the likelihood of such shifts is
small. The latter is the usual condition that faces us in the hospital
field, but though discouraging, the situation is by no means hopeless.
In place of competitive forces working to induce change on the supply
side pressures are arising from the demand side, i.e. from the
consumers or from those who pay for the consumers out of taxes
or insurance funds.

A widespread attack is being mounted, especially on hospital
hyperinflation, but it would be illusory to achieve a deceleration in

---

*See Chapter 2, p. 17.

the rate of price increases, or even an absolute lowering of prices
at the expense of reductions in quality and the number of services
offered or by increasing hospital deficits. What is needed are
techniques to achieve cost reduction while maintaining or even
improving the quantity and quality of health services—in this case
of hospital-produced health services.

Fortunately, even in the profit sector, as Leibenstein has
observed: "Empirical studies show that large cost reductions [can]
come from such activities as: simple reorganizations of the productive process, e.g. plant layout reorganization, materials handling,
waste controls, work methods, and payment by results."[2] To these
measures may be added improved on-the-job training, better
allocation, and supervision of personnel.

Approaches to and specific techniques of intrahospital cost
reduction may be discussed under a twofold classification—those
stemming primarily from endogenous efforts and those arising
primarily from exogenous sources, with some inevitable overlapping
areas.

To provide a focus for our discussion and in to avoid gener-
alizations and not-too-useful policy prescriptions based on them, we
present in Table 4.1 the departmental breakdown of the cost per
inpatient day of a fairly large (829 bed), voluntary, general hospital
in the Washington, D.C. area. This same hospital was featured in
a New York Times article* as the only large general hospital that
had reduced its charges in recent years. The average daily charge
was reduced in two steps from $120 per day to $117 and to $109 over
the period July 5 to September 15, 1971. In addition to a large
infusion of Medicaid funds that "covers the costs of services to the
poor but no more," the administrator listed the following "efficiencies"
responsible for controlling costs:

Giving incentive bonuses of up to $100 to employees who act
either to increase efficiency or to control costs.

Reducing overtime payment to employees from five percent of
the payroll to three percent.

Discharging patients earlier in the day when possible, thus
reducing unnecessary meals and spreading the housekeeping load
more evenly.

Ordering fewer duplicate laboratory tests once a person has
been admitted and been given an initial group of tests.

Purchasing cheaper drugs that are sold under their chemical
rather than their brand names.

---

*The New York Times, Sept. 15, 1971, p. 40.

TABLE 4.1

Cost Per Inpatient Day, Washington
Hospital Center, Washington, D.C., 1969

	Cost in Dollars	Percent of Total
Employee health and welfare	1.55	2
Administrative:		
Personnel administration		
General management		
Purchasing		
General accounting and data processing	12.42	13
Admitting department		
Development		
Volunteers		
Insurance malpractice		
Insurance general		
Plant operation	4.65	5
Laundry	1.51	2
Housekeeping	3.21	3
Pharmaceutical	2.97	3
Sterile supplies	1.35	1
Nursing service	23.20	25
Social service	.21	*
Medical records	1.77	2
Dietary	5.79	6
Nursing education	1.89	2
Interns and residents	4.29	5
Operating rooms	5.86	6
Delivery rooms	1.32	1
Anesthesia	3.57	4
Radiology	4.95	5
Laboratory	6.74	7
Intravenous solution	2.11	2
All other professional departments	3.62	4
Total	92.98	100[†]

*Less than one percent.
[†]May not add to 100 due to rounding.

Source: Testimony of Jose Blanco, Jr., Controller and Assistant Administrator, Washington Hospital Center, in, "High Cost of Hospitalization", Senate Hearings, 91st Congress, 2nd Session p.81., 1970.

Increasing the occupancy rate of the center's 845 beds to 83 percent from 82.

Giving daily baths to patients throughout the day, rather than only in the morning, thus spreading the nursing duties.

A key factor in keeping costs down was cooperation by the doctors.

The use of broad functional groupings that cut across departmental lines indicated that approximately 70 percent of the total cost was represented by salaries and wages. Using additional data provided in U.S. Senate testimony, we have calculated that 17 percent went for supplies, seven percent for a miscellaneous category,* and six percent for prospective depreciation. Obviously any program of meaningful cost reduction should concentrate on the largest of these elements—wages and salaries—with the "supplies" category receiving secondary attention.

Using a specific departmental breakdown, we note that nursing service, with 25 percent of the total, is by far the largest cost generator. Administrative departments rank second with 13 percent. The remaining departments are dispersed rather evenly within a one-six percent range. These data provide only a rough guide to the allocation of hospital cost-reducing efforts because this kind of cost analysis tells us nothing about the efficiency with which each department performs.

I have demonstrated elsewhere[3] that a more rational allocation of nursing personnel, utilizing all of the skills from those of the RN to aides would result not only in a saving of more than 25 percent in nursing expenses but an increase in available professional time as well. The twin goals of cost saving and quality improvement could thus be simultaneously achieved. The same principles of rational manpower utilization, moreover, might be applied in most of the other departments with the expectation of similar results. On this basis alone, before improvements in productivity per worker and before the substitution of capital for labor, the total wage and salary bill could be reduced. When the two other elements are added, the potential for reduction in cost per patient day must be judged to be of considerable magnitude. The question we wish to raise here, however, is: How can we induce the individual hospital manager to allocate his manpower rationally? The obvious answers are that he must first desire to reduce costs and second have the authority to overrule, in the above instance, the supervisor of the nursing department as well as the chief of the medical departments. His desire to

---

*Using the specific departmental breakdown, contractual obligations, fees, utilities, and maintenance.

reduce costs might stem—apart from the pride of craftsmanship—from the financial constraint of the prospective daily rate of care set by a reimbursement formula, of which more will be said below. Centering greater authority in the hands of the administrator is a problem that I leave to organizational theorists. Union-induced wage increases might also have a "shock effect" on administrators, forcing them to substitute less costly workers for more costly ones where possible. As I indicated in the article cited: "In order for us to realize these cost and efficiency savings we must strive to eliminate the 'demilitarized zones' that now exist between health occupations. This requires, among other things, a thoroughgoing review of licensure and certification requirements and a serious attempt to ease interstate mobility of workers through broadened reciprocity arrangements."[4]

It is gratifying to note that progress is being made in some of these areas. Walter McNerney, President of Blue Cross, has reported: "In Southern California, under CASH—Commission for Administrative Services in Hospitals . . . 90 hospitals are finding many new ways to improve services to the point where they expect to save a total of from 12 million to 16 million dollars annually. Following CASH suggestions, some hospitals now show a more than 20 percent improvement in the utilization of nursing personnel based on carefully formulated work standards and intense in-service education."[5] We should point out, however, that the improvements were brought about by "suggestions" rather than by imperatives, and also that 90 hospitals represent a small proportion of the more than 7,000 hospitals in the country.

It should have been stated at the outset perhaps that the time horizon within which all of the efficiency considerations are discussed is short-run. We are concerned, that is, with what steps an individual institution can take to promote operational efficiency with its existing hospital plant. This, of course, sets a basic constraint on ability to implement desired change. In the longer run this constraint is removed, opening up possibilities of a new plant that is architecturally sound and functionally flexible and will provide an environment more conducive to the efficient production of high-quality hospital services.

Even with the existing plant, however, there is much that can be done. In an interesting report on European efforts to promote hospital efficiency, the following time and cost savings estimates derived from centralization of auxiliary services and from work simplification and modernization were cited:

> Centralization of dishwashing by utilizing efficient
> dishwashing machines—time saving up to 80% and
> saving of operational costs up to 40%;

Central bed preparation at the time of change of
patients (including disinfection)—time saving up
to 20% and saving of operational costs up to 10%:

Centralization of cleaning and sterilizing of instru-
ments, syringes, and nursing equipment (within the
central sterilization)—time saving up to 30% and
saving of operational costs up to 20%;

Setting up of a central and if necessary [a] mech-
anized and automatic transport and communication
service—saving of time and operational costs up
to 60%;

Centralization of all operation theatres in one
central operation department—savings of rooms,
equipment, and supply up to 20% and savings of
operational costs up to 10%;

Centralization of equipment for X-ray diagnostics
of all medical specialties of the hospital in coordination with the automation of film processing,
film labelling, case transport—savings of room,
equipment and supply, and operational costs up to
10%;

Centralization of typing services in connection with
direct-dictating installations and centralization of
the files . . . , central transport services, and
pneumatic tube system—operational savings up
to 10%;

Rationalization of food distribution by means of
heating trolley system or tray system—time saving
up to 40% and saving of operational costs up to 20%;

Rationalization of writing work at the ward units by
utilization of reproduction procedures as well as by
means of utilization of uniform and expedient forms—
time and operational costs saving up to 20%;

Employment of film processing machines in the X-ray
department—time and operational costs saving up
to 10%;

> Improvement and rationalization of the booking tech-
> niques by means of booking machines, punch card system,
> or electronic data processing—savings of operational
> costs up to 15%;
>
> Expediently worked out forms for the admission — savings
> of operational costs up to 10%;
>
> Employment of labor-saving equipment in the laundry —
> time and operational cost savings up to 15%. . . .[6]

In addition to these techniques, the same report referred,
without specific cost-reduction estimates, to such factors as reduction
of working distances in areas other than those mentioned above, more
rational labor allocation, new organizational structure of the ward
area, over-all systems planning, use of electronic data processing,
the seven-day week, and several interhospital proposals that will be
discussed below.

It is interesting and significant, I think, that all of these
proposals, with the possible exception of those concerning interhospital
cooperation, involve activities that are to be undertaken within the
hospital. As modern a ring as they have, none of them concerns the
potential for cost reduction arising from the contracting out of
certain functions to external service firms. This reflects an
autarchical bias on the part of hospital administrators, i.e. toward
retaining control over all possible activities and avoiding dependence
on outside firms. There are, of course, some justifiable bases for
this attitude including the desire to prevent infections from coming
in or going out and the avoidance of interruptions of vital services
like food supply because of strikes or other events. In discussing
this problem elsewhere I have indicated that in a modern economy
such fears are probably exaggerated and that the practical benefits
to be derived from contracting out—in terms of both cost reduction
and of quality gains—can be significant.[7]

Now these and many other possible suggestions for promoting
cost and physical efficiency within the hospital are not entirely novel.
Indeed, hospitals appear to have been one of the first areas of
experimentation with what is called early "Taylorism." For example,
"The principles of Scientific Management, originated by Frederick
W. Taylor toward the end of the nineteenth century, were soon
applied in hospitals by Frank B. Gilbreth, who introduced motion
economy in several areas, including the surgical suite."[8] The
proliferation of industrial or management engineering groups
specializing in hospitals, however, is a product of the last two
decades. A brief compilation of such agencies would include:

The AHA, with its affiliated society, the Hospital Management Systems
Society, the Medical Division of the Operations Research Society of
America, the Hospital Division of the American Institute of Industrial
Engineers, the American Association of Hospital Consultants, the
American College of Hospital Administrators, Blue Cross, the
federal Hill-Burton Agency, specialized independent hospital consulting
groups, the management services divisions of health planning councils,
and state and local hospital associations. Two of the most important
continuing sources of information in this area are the Hospital
Administrative Services publications of the AHA and the PAS Reporter,
issued by the Commission on Professional and Hospital Activities
of Ann Arbor, Michigan. (The CASH group of Southern California
was referred to earlier.)

One would have to conclude, even on the basis of this incomplete
listing, that there is no dearth of advisors or of advice in the hospital
field. To this writer, and I'm certain to many hospital administrators
as well, it appears that there is an overabundance of data, that the
data are not always relevant, that their interpretation and presentation
are often faulty and that little is suggested as to methods for imple-
menting the findings and conclusions of consultants, even when
something constructive issues from the lengthy, often costly "studies."

To illustrate, the following table concerning the median hospital
stay for patients with an episode of acute coronary occlusion appeared
in one of the issues of the Record, a publication of the Commission
on Professional and Hospital Activities.

Even to one not trained in medicine it is obvious that the length
of hospital stay reflects the severity of the illness, the age, sex and
general disposition of the patient, medical complications and in some
cases the type of insurance coverage, conditions in the home, and
other factors. Variations in length of stay for any illness, therefore,
are to be expected. What appear as unusual variations to the authors
of the tabulation turn out, on closer inspection, to reveal remarkable
uniformity in median stays for coronary occlusion. For example,
the ranges of medians by hospital size starting with small hospitals
are 21, 19, 21, and 22 respectively. Even more remarkable is the
uniformity shown by the median of the medians. Half of all patients
with coronary occlusion in any hospital in North America, for
example, are almost certain to have a hospital stay of 21 days.

If this kind of distribution, suitably adjusted, is representative
of hospital stays for other illnesses, it would indicate that a good
deal of the effort now devoted to mitigating hospital cost by controlling
length of stay is wasted. More attention should be devoted to the
efficiency, in both physical and money terms, with which patient days
are in fact produced. It also suggests that proposed reimbursement
schemes that seek to vary payment by average (median) length of stay
will result in almost similar payments to all hospitals and will not

TABLE 4.2

Median Stay

Hospital Size	Number of Hospitals	Lowest Median	Median of Medians	Highest Median
Small	30	8	20	29
Medium small	56	11	21	30
Medium large	67	11	22	32
Large	67	12	22	34

Of the 30 small hospitals the median of medians
is twenty days. Yet there is at least one hospital
in the group that discharged half of its patients
on the eighth day or before and another that had
not discharged half its patients until the twenty-
ninth day. This highest median is more than a
threefold difference over the lowest. In the other
groups the highest medians are not quite three
times as great as the lowest.

All of the hospitals with lowest medians are
located west of the Mississippi River. Seven
hospitals have the highest medians; four of these
are Canadian and five are east of the Mississippi.
One of the hospitals with a highest median is in
the same state as a hospital with a lowest median.

Source: "High Cost of Hospitalization," Hearings Before the
Subcommittee on Antitrust and Monopoly, February and May 1970,
p. 511.

accomplish their objectives of rewarding "efficient" hospitals and
penalizing the "inefficient" ones—assuming that the latter are
socially desirable goals.

Let us pursue somewhat further this question of the relationship
between reimbursement techniques and efficiency. We noted earlier
in this work that third party payers—chiefly Blue Cross, commercial
insurers, and government—now account for at least 75 percent of
hospital operating income. Such groups, especially Blue Cross
because of its dominant position, are therefore in a position to use
their financial leverage to promote hospital efficiency. It has instead

been charged, with considerable supporting evidence, that the "Blues"
appear to have entered pacts of mutual solvency with hospitals and
have merely acted as accomplices in the cost "pass-through" pricing
practices of hospitals.[9] Edward M. Kaitz for example, has charged
more specifically that Blue Cross has contributed to hospital inefficiency by encouraging needless admissions and prolonged stays;
by adjusting reimbursement rates upward even though the increase
in average cost per day might have stemmed solely from a decrease
in occupancy rate; by distorting internal resource allocation through
encouragement of unneeded ancillary services and discouragement
of needed outpatient services; and by reimbursing automatically any
expansion of plant, facilities, and personnel.[10] Kaitz sums up his
case as follows:

> . . . [T]he study has shown that the cost-based third-
> party payment system has, all other forces being
> held constant, been a key force motivating the steady
> and inordinate increase in hospital costs in the past
> twenty years. It has helped to increase costs by
> removing a substantial portion of the business risk
> in hospital operations while failing to provide either
> an incentive for efficient production of medical care
> or a penalty for inefficient production.[11]

Additional evidence of the rather passive role of Blue Cross
vis-a-vis hospitals was provided in the Senate Hearings on "The
High Cost of Hospitalization," previously cited. The testimony of
James C. Brown, senior vice president of Blue Cross of Southern
California indicated that in a universe of 310 general hospitals and
400 extended-care facilities with a total of 150,000 admissions during
1969, 99.4 percent of the admissions were approved for payment.[12]
While the present writer agrees generally with these accusations
against the "Blues" and the "for-profit" health insurance carriers,
and, in fact, further questions whether the principle of "actuarial
soundness" should have any place at all in health care, some incon-
sistencies and analytical faults in Kaitz's presentation should be
indicated. He states for instance, that the ". . .Blue Cross System
was used only to determine the floor for prices. The final decision
on prices was made after placing a few telephone calls to neighboring
hospitals to ascertain that the retail price for ancillary services was
consistent with area-wide pricing."[13] He also indicates that price
appears to be determined by an informal consensus technique based
on "what the other fellow is doing. . . ."[14] Clearly, if these statements
hold, interhospital collusion is as much to be blamed for high prices
as is Blue Cross. With respect to the "misallocation" of resources

in favor of ancillary services charged by Kaitz he states that ". . .
ancillary services are regarded as indicators of the technological
competence and the quality of care provided by a hospital. . ."[15]
Blue Cross should not be faulted, however, for inducing hospitals
to upgrade their quality, surely a socially desirable goal. Kaitz
makes much of the point that Blue Cross and government reimbursement rates are lower than those paid by self-paying patients: "The
effect of granting a cost advantage to the state and Blue Cross is to
increase the price that must be charged the non-Blue Cross and
non-welfare consumer. Thus the 'retail price' for hospital care
must be set higher than it would be set if no one were granted a
price advantage."[16] This statement would be true only if average
costs were constant or even increased with respect to output
(occupancy rate). If, as a good deal of evidence suggests (see chapters
and 1 and 2), average costs decline over some range of output "bulk
purchases" inducing higher occupancy rates might actually help reduce
average costs per day, not only justifying lower rates for themselves
but also possibly lowering rates even for direct-pay patients.

In Appendix C of <u>The Demand Determinant Role of the Physician</u>
Kaitz points up an important locus of cost generation in the hospital—
the physician. In rural and suburban areas especially, the physician,
or a small group of physicians play a crucial role in hospital building
and/or expansion. In all hospitals generally, as Kaitz indicates, the
physician orders about 80 percent of the dollar value of services
rendered an individual patient. Certainly, evaluating and modifying
physician behavior through such devices as medical audits and peer
review appear to be fruitful areas in which to achieve intrahospital
cost reductions.

The 1970 Member Hospital Reimbursement Formula of the
Associated Hospital Service of New York (Blue Cross)[17] is an
attempt to meet the various critiques of reimbursement mentioned
above and is also an attempt to conform to New York's 1969 Cost
Control Law which

> mandates specifically that in providing for the efficient
> production of hospital service, account must be taken of:
> (1) the elements of costs, (2) geographical differentials
> in elements of costs, (3) economic factors in the hospital's
> area, (4) rates of increase or decrease of the area's
> economy, (5) costs of hospitals of comparable size,
> (6) need for incentives to improve services and encourage
> economy, (7) adapting joint central services when appro-
> riate, (8) excluding research and educational costs.[18]

The major new approach embodied in the AHS document (page references in parentheses) is the use of prospective as opposed to retrospective reimbursement. Instead of paying hospitals for their reported costs as in the past the new formula sets limits to cost increases based on estimated changes in operating costs of comparable hospitals as well as on the "projected movement" of "selected indices" deemed to be reflective of those elements of the hospital economy comparable to the general economy in the coming 12-month period.[19] The new formula confines capital cost reimbursement only to those facilities that have been approved by an areawide planning group (11). It provides productivity incentive payment "to hospitals acquiring capital assets designed to reduce labor costs by increasing the efficient production of hospital services (16). It contains a utilization incentive "in order to give recognition to the importance of optimum use of expensive inpatient hospital facilities and to stimulate continual attention to limiting length of stay to that period appropriate and proper to patient care. . . ." (19). It attempts to encourage ambulatory services by providing for a "Community Service Factor" (22). It eliminates from allowable operating costs certain research and educational expenses as well as other non-patient associated hospital activities (23 and 25). It eliminates excess costs caused by under-utilized services (30). It sets payment rates for ambulatory services. This formula also goes beyond previous ones in demanding uniform reporting through its auditing requirements and by imposing penalties for late reports.

This new reimbursement formula, in short, represents in many respects a radical departure from prior ones. Whether its various incentives are strong enough to rectify inefficiencies and thereby limit cost increases remains to be seen. Some progress, however, has already been recorded. Medicaid reimbursement rates for the first half of 1971, which are based on a formula similar to the 1970 AHS rate just described, rose by 12.9 percent, some six percent less than the rates that should have prevailed to the enactment of the New York State Cost Control Law.[20]

While such legal measures might be effective in reducing the rate of growth of hospital inflation, the more basic problem is reducing absolute levels of hospital costs. Within the existing hospital control framework, the objective of cost reduction would appear to be pursued efficaciously along two routes—the provision of incentives to hospital personnel, including physicians, to achieve large productivity increases and the achievement of a more rational division of labor among hospitals. The first of these will be discussed briefly at this point, the second in the following chapter.

In the first chapter we noted that most hospitals are either governmental or nongovernmental. The term "voluntary" does not mean that garden variety economic motives of hospital employees

are nonoperative or only mildly operative. Growing militancy on
economic issues, rising unionization, and various other work actions
attest to the contrary. While the psychic income of hospital workers
probably exceeds that of most other groups, it is the reality of the
relatively low incomes that predominates. Periodic disclosures of
the high income of some health professionals, like the recent
report that physicians' current median incomes are $40,550.00,[21]
increase the sense of relative deprivation of hospital workers
and perhaps even of hospital-based physicians (pathologists, radiologists, and anesthesiologists excepted). In view of these factors,
we concur fully with Gilpatrick's and Corliss' statement that
"implementation of a manpower structure in hospitals to achieve
the goals described [motivation, efficiency, etc.] must be derived
from a self-propelled system in which the goals are achieved by
the parties following their own interests and not by the exhortation
to sacrifice them."[22]

Though not yet widespread, experiments in providing usually
deferred monetary incentives to increase the efficiency of hospital
employees are under way at several hospitals in the U.S. In what
has been described as "the first attempt to successfully apply the
principles of total systems incentives to a nonprofit, private hospital
enterprise."[23] J. J. Jehring evaluates the first five years of a
profit-sharing program in effect at the Long Beach Memorial
Hospital, California. There are some interesting and, it would
appear, widely applicable features of its so-called MERIT (Memorial
Employees Retirement Incentive Trust) Plan. First, incentives to
efficiency are group or departmental in scope rather than directed
at the individual worker—recognition of the fact that in many hospital
structures the contribution of individual workers is difficult, if not
impossible to measure. Second, "profits" that are shared are in
reality cost savings in a given time period relative to that of a
previous three-year period and realized by a department in discharging
its responsibilities. Third, employees are not held responsible for
activities over which they have little or no control, such as depreciation and interest expense. Finally, gains are tax exempt and are
placed in a trust that is managed by professional investment personnel.
The entire plan is coordinated with a work simplification program.

The results of the program have been impressive. There has
been a reduction in personnel turnover, more efficient utilization of
nursing service, better collection of accounts, improved efficiency
in central services, and a lower cost-per-patient day than in comparable hospitals in the same area. Most of the improvement,
according to Jehring, came about "through motivating employees in
the direction of making improvements and eliminating waste."[24]
As one employee stated in an interview with the hospital's executive

committee: "People are cost conscious because [the Plan]—it increases understanding between what they do and what they say; nurses think twice about costs."[25] In the Baptist Hospital at Pensacola, Florida, where a similar system was introduced, the administrator stated:

> Because of incentives we have had to become profit
> and productivity minded at all levels of our organi-
> zation. We began using unit cost rather than gross
> figures to measure results. This gave us something
> we could talk about to individual employees, some-
> thing they would understand. We looked at staffing
> levels and began to relate them to some unit or pro-
> ductivity such as how many man hours per laboratory
> procedure. Another thing we have had to do because
> of incentives is to define the product each area or
> department was producing.

and further:

> We have forced ourselves to set both long-range and
> short-range goals from a management standpoint as
> well as employee standpoint. We found as we pro-
> gressed that we needed additional knowledge about
> what makes people work, and so all of us have had to
> look at our organization in an entirely different way.
> This had been very healthy for us.[26]

That a carrot-sans-stick approach can increase employee productivity is probably correct. One must not, however, expect too much from such techniques. As Schiel has pointed out, "incentives are not substitutes for good training, good selection, basic salary plans, or a good work atmosphere in any sense of the word. They are the icing on the cake rather than the cake itself."[27]

Clearly, we have not exhausted the sources of intrahospital cost reduction potential and of the means for their achievement. In a dynamic economy the search for optimum combinations of input factors is a continuous one. In the hospital economy the discovery of such techniques is a necessary but insufficient condition for their application. The search for incentives to perform appropriate to a health situation is of equal importance.

The spatial and functional distributions of American hospitals have been influenced by a variety of factors including population movement, availability of capital, location of physicians, governmental requirements, and historical accident. These factors have operated with different intensity with the result that existing distributions are not optimal from either a demographic or a functional point of view. Prior to the passage of the Hill-Burton Law in 1946, as Anne Somers has observed, "[a]ny hospital that could raise the money could build, expand, contract or otherwise alter the hospital resources of the community without clearance from any public body."[1]

Moreover, the existence of three different types of control—voluntary, proprietary, and governmental (all levels)—precluded the kind of coordination of facilities that would be possible, for instance, under a nationalized health service. If market forces alone were operative one might expect to find that hospitals functioning under deficit conditions would close their doors and relocate to more lucrative areas, i.e. cater to higher income groups. While such movement might result in an economically optimal distribution—and in fact proprietary hospital and physician location appears to follow this pattern—it need not result in a socially optimum one. When, therefore, one takes into account the relative immobility of fixed hospital plants, the many types of health manpower, and the fact that deficits are frequently made up by community appeals, welfare funds, or some other means, the factors that might be expected to generate economically predictable locational patterns in fact fall short of doing so. That they are not completely inoperative, however, is demonstrated by the dearth of hospitals in many rural areas and the abandonment or critical understaffing of pre-existing hospitals in inner city areas. The relative lack of nursing homes, of geriatric and chronic disease hospitals, and of rehabilitation facilities also attests to the influence of economic factors. Of course, medical and social factors are likewise heavily involved. David D. Rutstein has noted: "Our general hospitals, devoted mainly to the care of acute short-term illness, are symptomatic of the episodic nature and lack of continuity that pervades our medical care. Moreover, the discharge of chronically ill patients from the general hospitals to the miserably inadequate care in nursing homes re-emphasizes our lack of real concern for the chronically ill and aged."[2]

In the previously cited Report of the European Health Committee, a rational approach—both medically and economically—to the distribution of hospital facilities was set forth and, because of the sharp contrast it offers to the American picture, merits citation at some length:

> An analysis of the demand for in-patient hospital services shows that the total demand for hospital beds is far from being uniformly distributed over the various medical specialties and differs greatly from one to another. Almost three quarters of the total demand (approx: 70%) are required by the main services: surgery and internal medicine (including infectious diseases) and gynaecology/ obstetrics; further approx. 17% by the service paediatrics, throat, nose, ear and eye diseases; the remaining approx. 13% by the other services. (Not taken into consideration here are the special disciplines such as psychiatry, tuberculosis, crippled patients etc., with long-staying patients.) However, also within the various specialties there exists for certain treatments a great demand and again for other treatments only a small demand for hospital beds. It is also a fact that for an efficient specialised service, for medical and nursing reasons (necessary medical routine) as well as for economic reasons (favourable personnel situation, economic utilisation of space equipment and supply), the number of beds of a medical specialty must not fall below a certain inferior limit. From this point of view, the varying high demand for special hospital beds as well as the minimum size of a medical specialty make it appear necessary to graduate the total number of beds available within the general in-patient hospital services according to the several stages of requirements. On a lower level hospital beds must be available for the kind of treatment which can be spread over a large region (basic service). Moreover, on a central level those hospital beds must be

available that do not allow a widespread dispersal to all
general hospitals (regular service). Finally, on the
upper level special beds and special equipment have to
be provided which are used relatively seldom and which,
therefore, for medical, nursing and economic reasons
have to be centralised (central service). The density of
this network of general hospitals with different requirements has to be in conformity with the population density
and traffic connections. It is, of course, obvious that in
less densely populated regions with bad traffic connections
this basic set-up has to be modified accordingly. However,
there is much to be said for rather putting up with longer
and more complicated transports of patients than to
decentralise certain special beds and special services in
a way which cannot be justified either from the medical
and nursing point of view or from the economic side.
[Original spelling and usage.][3]

Citing the increasing complexity of modern diagnostic and
therapeutic procedures and the potential economies of scale of larger
hospitals or of individual departments, the same report recommended
the centralization of services for a group of hospitals. Among the
most important of such shared services recommended are:

1a) Joint utilisation of treatment facilities: In the
medical field the further development of diagnostic and
therapy involves a continuous specialisation. However,
the sensible employment of specialists and special equipment demands a respectively larger capacity of per-
formances which is no longer available in the individual
hospital but only in collaboration with several hospitals.
Practical experience offers two possibilities of collaboration: each hospital specialises on special per-
formances (example: specialisation of the laboratories
or special examination groups) or else several hospitals
run jointly special installations and equipment (example:
pathology).
1b) Joint utilisation of supply facilities: Examples:
Centralisation of sterilisation work for several hospitals;
central pharmacy; central laundry; central cooking
factory for deep frozen ready-made food; central cleaning
and technical services.
1c) Joint utilisation of administrative facilities:
Examples: Joint procurement organisation (central
purchase and central stock-keeping); uniform

> arrangement of forms and joint printing of the forms;
> central bed assessment; joint emergency services
> (alternating from hospital to hospital); standardising of
> the accounting and joint utilisation of electronic data
> processing centre.[4]

In support of recommendation 1a) above, a recent report by a
surgery study group indicated that " . . . to maintain standards and
function efficiently, hospital centers doing open-heart surgery should
have a case demand requiring four to six operations a week, or about
200 annually. But . . . a 1969 survey showed [that] only 15 of 360
hospitals studied performed the recommended number of open-heart
procedures."[5]

In 1966 Mark Blumberg cited some attempts by groups of
hospitals to rationalize their treatment facilities, for example:

> The Greater Detroit Area Hospital Council has been quite
> successful in persuading several hospitals to merge their
> obstetric facilities in one institution rather than to operate
> autonomous services . . . A similar program is under
> way to merge pediatric facilities.

Blumberg added:

> In Passaic County, New Jersey, six voluntary hospitals
> have worked out a cooperative arrangement whereby
> only one of them has the following types of services:
> open-heart surgery, iron lung, artificial kidney,
> electronic aphalogram, clinic for retarded children,
> poison control center, rehabilitation physiotherapy,
> and cobalt treatment.[6]

If the report on underutilization of open-heart surgery facilities
noted above is representative the case of coordination reported by
Blumberg was evidently not widely imitated. There are also some
examples in his study of the joint utilization of supply and administrative facilities (b and c above), but the number of instances reported
is small. On the other hand, notes Blumberg, "[w]e find a great deal
of cooperation among hospitals in such areas as collections of unpaid
bills and fund raising."[7] Needless to say, this latter type of cooperation, as well as the informal cooperation on price setting noted
earlier, is not calculated to bring rationalization, efficiency, or cost
abatement to the hospital arena.

Beginning in the 1960s and continuing into the 1970s with great
frequency, serious students of the health scene as well as _ad hoc_

commissions began to pay increasing attention to the hospital as part
of a system. It became obvious that no matter how well managed
single institutions could do little to affect costs and the underlying
major health problems that are both the cause and effect of cost
escalation: fragmentation of care, maldistribution and misallocation
of facilities and manpower, extreme duplication, among other factors.
Similarly, the Report of the [New York] Governor's Committee on
Hospital Costs[8] noted that " . . . hospitals, accustomed and organized
to act intramurally have thus far not been able to achieve many of
the economies and improvements that require extramural action."[9]

There can be little doubt, therefore, that one of the major
health planning tasks of the 1970s will be the de-autonomization of
hospitals and health facilities generally. The committee went even
further:

> To utilize hospitals more fully would require definitive
> action to close down institutions that no longer should
> be operated; to convert some to other needed purposes;
> to consolidate services and hospitals; to coordinate
> programs; to build more flexible facilities that would
> permit a higher level of occupancy—in brief, to
> regionalize and rationalize more fully the plant and
> operations of hospitals in New York State: to decide on
> the kind of hospital system that is needed—one that can
> operate more efficiently—and to proceed to establish
> it.[10]

Although the report was concerned with New York state hospitals, its conclusions in our view are more widely applicable and, in
fact, might be more appropriate to other parts of the nation where
counterparts of the Metcalf-McCloskey Act of 1964, the Folsom Act
of 1965, and the New York Cost Control Act of 1969 do not yet exist.

Allusion was made in the above quotation to regionalization.
In their comprehensive evaluation of a regional health program in
Michigan, McNerney and Riedel, quoting from an earlier work of
Donabedian and Axelrod, define the term as follows:

> In its pure form, this concept [health regionalization]
> envisages the unified planning of a functionally differ-
> entiated and carefully coordinated system of hospitals
> serving an entire geographic region demarcated, not by
> narrow political boundaires, but according to established
> patterns of seeking and providing medical care in a
> manner analogous to trading areas. Under such a plan,
> standards of medical care could be considerably

improved throughout the region, without costly duplication or inefficient development of scarce resources
and skills. There would be established appropriately
located central or base hospitals to which other smaller
hospitals in the region would turn for help and advice.
The central hospital would, in turn, assume considerable
responsibility for supporting continuing professional
education and medical and allied services in the hospitals
associated with it.[11]

The similarity between this regional concept and that of the
European Public Health Committee report cited earlier is, of course,
very great. The problem, obviously, is not a conceptual one but
rather one of removing the barriers to regionalization that, according
to McNerney and Riedel, include " . . . a strongly rooted concept of
local autonomy and a corollary apprehension of direct governmental
intervention."[12] Both of these forces, one might observe, appear to
be accomodated in the education field in which the local high school
or state university unit to which deep pride is often attached are
nevertheless governmentally financed and state supervised institutions.
This analogy holds in those cases in which the local health facility
is indeed a municipal or county institution, although it must be
admitted that underfinanced and undermanned governmental hospitals
gradually lose whatever local pride that might once have existed.
The health education analogy is tenuous, however, because so large
a proportion of hospitals and even more of hospital beds* are nongovernmental and not-for-profit types. The "voluntary" appellation
provides added layers of resistance to the necessary process of
de-autonomization. When one looks behind nomenclature, however,
the realities of the high cost of autonomy in both monetary and health
terms and the financial dependence of nominally "independent" units
on government funds (either directly via capital and operating costs
or indirectly via tax exemptions) become apparent. One recent
investigative group put the matter forcefully:

The Task Force believes that the day is past when doctors
and hospital administrators and trustees and their as-
sociates may rely on their own judgements of how they
can best distribute all the skills and resources at their
disposal to what they see as the greatest advantage for the
people they think they should be serving. The resources
today in substantial part are public or community

---

*See Table 1.3.

resources, not excluding physicians trained largely at public expense; and their allocation and conditions of aid are thus a public concern. The escalation from individual need to community crisis to public funding to public decision making is the choreography of social action in a democratic society.[13]

In addition to these arguments, the case for social control in the health field is strengthened further when one considers the externalities involved; it should be recognized that the individual purchase or receipt of health care provides social as well as individual benefits (most directly in the case of individual immunization against communicable disease). The larger the proportion of social benefits, the stronger is the case for governmental intervention to maximize social welfare. Given the arguments presented, it is difficult not to accept the principle of social intervention with respect to the allocation and utilization of resources in the hospital and health field. Indeed, the United States is unique among the world's nations in that the principle is still subject to debate. The kind of social intervention we have had to date, however—e.g. Medicare and Medicaid—has been necessitated by the high cost of hospitalization and the consequent denial of health services to large portions of the community. They have been stopgap financial measures and apart from setting certain minimal standards for health facilities have done little to promote the kind of systematic coordination we have been discussing.[14] Neither of these measures, it should be added, has contributed to cost abatement. Quite the contrary, by increasing effective demand while leaving supply unaffected, they have provided further impetus to hospital cost inflation.

It now appears that a combination of financing and control-coordinating mechanisms is required if the hospital and health system is to meet the increasing demands upon it efficiently. One need not be doctrinaire, however, on choosing the means for achieving greater coordination and efficiency. A decree "nationalizing" all health care facilities—i.e., one converting all voluntary and proprietary (at book-value compensation) into governmentally owned facilities— would in all probability be counterproductive and would result in chaos for a long time. The wiser course would be to use appropriate legislative machinery, economic leverage, and other incentives to begin to shape the production and distribution of health services so as to reap the maximum benefits of a coordinated system without generating negative side effects. We cannot now perceive precisely what the contours of the system will ultimately resemble. While most professional health planners, for example, have an anti-proprietary bias, (in the health field the unrestrained profit motive

can be and often is most pernicious), it should be recognized that in
some areas of the country proprietary hospitals render a higher
quality of care at lower costs than do surrounding voluntary or
governmental institutions. This suggests that some proprietary
hospitals might be able to function as yard-sticks against which to
measure the quality and costs of "non-profit" institutions—reversing
the role that TVA plays in the mostly private electrical power
industry. The deterioration of many municipal, state, and county
hospitals* has already been defined, so one cannot determine merely
from the type of control the quality and quantity of health services
rendered. To spread my criticisms equally, it has been noted that
many voluntary hospitals appear to exist more to insure the high
incomes of referring physicians than to treat all who need care
according to the highest dictates and standards of medical practice.
The scandalous conditions of many proprietary "nursing homes"
alone need be mentioned to illustrate the point. These brief, not
unbiased, comments might serve to make us wary of a priori judgments
in this area.

Platitudinous as it may sound, one must agree with Anne R.
Somers' view, quoting McNerney, that what is needed is to ". . . provide
discipline to the system without smothering its initiative and
vitality."15

Restructuring of the hospital system can be accomplished by
a combination of the use of federal and state regulatory powers, an
appropriate system of financing of health services (a matter quite
different from a scheme of national health insurance) and, since the
latter will take many years to achieve, the current reimbursement
process to initiate movement. The existing status of hospital regulation has been comprehensively and lucidly reviewed by Anne R. Somers
in the book already cited. She traces the legal treatment of the hospital in common law and discusses recent decisions concerning tax
law, labor law, personnel and facility licensure, and the incentives
(or lack of them) to efficiency embodied in current and proposed
reimbursement schemes. Mrs. Somers' major emphasis is on how
the individual hospital's operations and standards are affected by
various kinds of uncoordinated regulation. She raises the question
of the treatment of the hospital industry as a public utility and rejects
it on the grounds that there exists no single pattern of public utility
regulation in this country that might serve as a model, that public
service commissions have too often served industries rather than

---

*See the author's chapter, "Capital Funding" in Urban Health
Services: The Case of New York, by Eli Ginzberg et al., (New York:
Columbia University Press, 1971).

the public, that, " . . . it would be administratively impossible to
regulate the hospital industry with its seven thousand separate units"
(215), that 85 percent of the units are nonprofit, and that the product
is highly individualized.[16] These arguments are not entirely convincing. The fact that we do not have a good model of public utility
regulation means that we can be all the more flexible in devising a
system that is most appropriate to the characteristics of the hospital
industry. The fact that public service commissions have not proved
adequate does not mean that they cannot under any circumstances
function effectively. The regulation of 7,000 units pales into in-
significance in comparison with government regulation in education,
in the setting and enforcement of minimum wage laws, in the coordination of global defense forces, and in the administration of the
social security laws, for example. Furthermore, regulation also
implies coordination and consolidation so that in place of 7,000
separate units, the focus of regulation might be 700 or even 70 regional
hospital systems. The fact that most of the units are nonprofit and
that therefore there are no "inordinate profits" to control is likewise
not a strong argument against regulation. Inordinate prices are just
as valid a reason for control as profits. As Clair Wilcox has pointed
out with respect to other utility services including gas, electricity,
and phones: "They are essentials bought continuously by many small
consumers. For them, the need is urgent and is not postponable.
And there are no acceptable alternatives. The buyers must meet the
seller's terms or go without. It is this that sets the public utilities
apart, explaining why regulation is required."[17] Finally, the notion
that the product is individualized appears to be irrelevant. The fact
that each child is different and learns in different ways and at different
rates does not preclude public regulation and ownership of schools.

It might very well be true, as Mrs. Somers suggests, that
"[t]o declare the hospital a public utility at this stage might have the
virtue of apparent simplicity, but it would be misleading. It would
simply substitute a slogan for the hard thinking that is required if
the present maze of public laws and regulations is to be rationalized
and systematized into something approaching a positive creation
policy. The net result of adopting the background slogan would almost
surely be negative."[18] On the other hand, by not adopting the
"slogan"—and more important the reality it connotes—some 40 years
ago when it was suggested by Rufus Rorem (208) the hospital "system"
was allowed to drift into its present unsatisfactory state. At some
point the issue must be faced directly. Whether we use the phrase
public utility or some other phrase such as "public service corpo-
ration" (208) is not as important as the recognition that over-all
public regulation is imminently required. It should also be pointed
out that public utility status and nationalization are not synonymous;

we have already indicated that the latter should not be first on the
agenda of public policy. Mrs. Somers' negative views regarding the
public utility approach and not the solution to the hospital malaise
results from her overly restrictive view of the concept.

We have so far discussed the broad outlines of what a rational
hospital system should resemble, suggesting that it might be con-
trolled and directed on the basis of some as yet imprecisely defined
public utility model. The Task Force on Medical and Related Problems
(hereafter the Task Force) to which we have referred has indicated
how the plan of reorganization might possibly begin. The first phase
of the plan would involve the recognition that the existing division
of labor in hospital facilities is suboptimal and that new functional
types are needed. The Task Force therefore recommended that
approximately five percent of federal Medicaid funds be appropriated
each year and with the cooperation of state and areawide health
planning agencies we should support such activities as:

> . . . development of organized primary health-care
> services in neighborhoods; development of services and
> resources which can serve as alternatives to inpatient
> hospital care, e.g. home health-care programs; improve-
> ments in utilization, efficiency and/or quality of existing
> health services directed to producing more and better
> health care; social and other outreach services which are
> an integral aspect of appropriate utilization of services;
> development of ways to link and relate new and existing
> health services with each other, aiming toward compre-
> hensive health-care systems in communities.[19]

Obviously portions of funds from other federal health programs
such as Medicare, Hill-Burton, Regional Medical, and Community
Mental Health should also be used to encourage such programs and,
when necessary, new funding sources could be created. The Secretary's Advisory Committee on Hospital Effectiveness (the Barr
Report) went a step further in recommending that "[w]here such
arrangements will assist the institutions in meeting the purposes of
the planned project, state health facilities licensing agencies shall
condition the approval of projects seeking federal funds on the
existence of formal contractual arrangements between institutions
for shared administration, medical staff appointments, and privileges,
services offered and facilities furnished."*

---

*"Report of Secretary's Advisory Committee on Hospital Effec-
tiveness," U.S. Department of Health, Education and Welfare (1968),
p. 13.

In addition to encouraging innovation by function, the Task Force also supported the concept of the Health Maintenance Organization (HMO) as a way of modifying the structure of health service delivery.[20] The basic concept of HMO is similar to such existing prepaid organizational plans as the Kaiser-Permanente and the Health Insurance Plan of New York. A detailed evaluation of such plans is beyond the scope of the present work. Suffice it to say, however, that such plans now involve a small proportion of the nation's physicians and other health manpower as well as small, selected proportions of the population, even though these plans have been operating for about a quarter of a century. Since they do represent a kernel of what a comprehensive health system should resemble they should, in my view, be encouraged.* We should not underestimate the massive incentives and the time required to create and expand HMOs, however. If these structures are found not to be yielding results, we should be prepared to abandon the effort in favor of a more thoroughgoing structural overhaul.

Since the locus of control over the health system now resides in the states rather than in the federal government—where, I believe, it ought to be if we are to ever devise a workable national system—plans for reform must concentrate on state health, education, social service, and insurance departments. The health portions of the latter three should be consolidated with the first to create one state health agency for the supervision and administration of health programs. Since many health problems cannot be confined to states' borders regional bodies** are needed to coordinate the activities of several states. Over-all supervision might be centered in a board of governors of a federal health system along the lines of the Federal Reserve. Reference to the latter model is not entirely inappropriate because it combines private and public sectors and operates in many areas by indirect rather than direct actions—administrative techniques well suited to the hospital area.[†]

----

*This would require the immediate, long overdue removal of all state legislative barriers to prepaid group practices.

**Not to be confused with the existing Regional Medical Program.

[†] I would suggest that unlike the Federal Reserve System, in which almost half of all banks are not members, membership in the proposed federal health system be made mandatory and that all health facilities be included. Some organic connection with the Department of HEW would also be required. Whether this requires federal incorporation of hospitals is a moot point. So long as there are uniform national standards that are enforced state incorporation might suffice.

A similar approach to the problem of restructuring was sketched out by Irving J. Lewis:

> The health establishment needs organizations that can plan and manage the delivery of health care at the community level with real authority. The precise nature of such a "community trustee" remains to be defined, but some of its desirable characteristics mix with strong consumer involvement; this may make health professionals uncomfortable but they will have to realize that they can no longer go it alone. It should be based on a principle of geographic responsibility and be strong enough to exact from the medical resources of its area—physicians, hospitals, and others—the performance of defined health-care functions. It should reflect at the local level a public-private, lay-professional alliance that reaches up to some form of health commission or board at the Federal level that can see the country's health needs as a whole.[21]

An integral part of a state health department restructured along the proposed lines would be a state health facility rate-setting commission that should be independent of existing state insurance departments and charged with establishing prices of health services. Such a commission was created by Massachusetts in 1968 and in New York in 1969 with the Cost Control Law. While it did not set up a separate commission the latter gave similar powers over hospital rates to the commissioner of insurance. Under the Massachusetts statute "[a]ll providers of health care doing business with the state government are required to provide the Commission with such data as it may request, to permit inspection of their books and, subject to the right of appeal, to accept payment at the rate established by the Commission."[22]

This writer would broaden the mandate to include all facilities, irrespective of whether they are doing business with the state, and would add unannounced medical quality audits to stipulated financial audits. Furthermore, as soon as a broadened and strengthened state health department is set up a moratorium on all facility construction should be declared. This would provide an opportunity to develop a complete inventory of state health facilities, along not only quantitative but functional and qualitative lines. Plans should be simultaneously drawn up to phase out duplicated facilities and to implement functional changes, i.e. perhaps converting small proprietary and voluntary hospitals into diagnostic or ambulatory facilities or into extended-care or geriatric units. At the expiration of the moratorium, no

application for construction should be passed unless it has met all
prior requirements of a comprehensive health planning group, a
constituent agency of the health department.*

The "rate setting" proposed here would not be an individual
hospital rate but rather, an area-wide, average rate. Since I cannot
envision a rational system that does not provide coverage for the
total population, for all health services, criteria other than existing
actuarial ones would have to be devised.†

In a recent study Anne R. Sommers made a case for the calculation
of a community average costs calculation that might be the basis for
community-wide rate setting. She wrote:

> With respect to hospital costs there are two basic facts
> that must be kept in mind if we are to come to grips with
> this seemingly intractable problem:
>   1. The more cooperative and successful a hospital
> is in limiting admission to serious cases, in holding
> lengthy stays down to the absolute minimum, and other-
> wise fulfilling the demands of the planners, the higher
> its per diem costs will inevitably go.
>   2. From the point of view of social accounting the
> only way this situation can be dealt with intelligently is
> to average the costs of this increasingly expensive,
> specialized institution with the less expensive satellite
> and affiliated institutions. If this were done, the inevitably
> high costs of the inpatient unit could be absorbed in total
> community costs just as the inevitably high costs of the
> hospital's intensive care unit are averaged in the costs
> of the institution as a whole. This is only possible
> however, in a system that is rationalized not only
> organizationally but financially.[23]

There can be little doubt that in order to implement such a
proposal, one must recognize, as Mrs. Somers has observed, that

---

*Depreciation allowances of hospitals would be funded and
pooled and placed under the control of the health department.

†I do not minimize the difficulties involved. From a technical
viewpoint, I am inclined to favor average over marginal cost pricing
since I do not think that hospital admissions should be determined
by the marginal cost-marginal revenue criterion but solely by the
criteria of bed availability and patient need. Moreover, in the presence
of considerable externalities, neither calculated marginal now
average costs are appropriate-"shadow" prices are more relevant.

"[t]he key to progress appears to lie in the increasing integration
or coordination of separate hospital, medical and other health care
costs into a single total community-wide accounting system."24

It should be emphasized that community-wide cost averaging
does not obviate the necessity of constant surveillance to increase
efficiency within institutions. In effect this over-all approach enables
us to deal with wide deviations from efficiency and quality norms in
a more rational manner than that permitted by current approaches,
which are couched in terms of "rewarding the efficient and penalizing
the inefficient institutions." The latter formula, which has been
offered as a substitute for full costs reimbursement, would only
exacerbate the situation by helping to make less efficient hospitals
still less efficient by denying them funds needed for improvement.
This hypothesis assumes that neither efficient nor inefficient institutions trade quality for efficiency. Given a systematic, i.e. community or area-wide orientation and average costing, it would behoove
state authorities to increase the flow of funds to inefficient hospitals
so that by attracting superior management talent, by automating, or
by other means, the inefficient hospital might be brought up to par.
Since the inefficient hospital is by definition a high-cost one, investing
in it to raise its efficiency level would lower its costs, therefore the
average costs for the system as a whole, other things being equal. If the
investment is of a nonrecurring nature, that is to say, if efficiency
can in fact be improved, its yield over time in terms of lowered cost
of services will far exceed costs.

All of these considerations must be taken apart from the economies that the system would realize by centralized purchasing, laundry,
laboratories and other factors. It is incredible to note, for example,
that so far as the present writer is aware, there exists no automated
central hospital bed reservation system on a community-wide basis
in the United States comparable, say, to seat reservations on air
lines or room reservations for many hotels and recreational events.
Undoubtedly the existing autonomy of hospitals combined with present
physician affiliation procedures militates against such a central
system.* Reforms in present practices whereby decisions are made

---

*An excellent example of the medical and economic benefits that
might be derived from centralizing certain functions as opposed to
performing them separately in each hospital was provided in an article
concerning the King County Central Blood Bank in Seattle. One central
facility supplies all of the blood needs for Seattle's 32 hospitals at a
cost that is " . . . at least half of what they are anywhere else" and
what is more important, at a minimal risk of the recipient's contracting hepatitis. (Cf. The New York Times, October 27, 1971.)

as to which patients go to which hospitals at what time are urgently required and are additional cogent reasons for substituting a large measure of social control for autonomy.

What place is there, then, for incentives and how can they be utilized in the social control framework outlined? My proposal would be to trade off some degree of autonomy for the individual institution in return for high quality care efficiently produced. That is to say, consonant with community service needs and plans, those institutions that are able to render high-quality, efficient services, would be entitled to some independent control over research programs, internal manpower distribution, some salary scales and other conditions of work.

In short, autonomy is a status that should be earned. It should not be viewed, as it is at present, as an inherent right of an institution but as a privilege to be won gradually through good works. The basic assumptions underlying this proposal are that some degree of autonomy is necessary for the preservation and promotion of a hospital's vitality and innovativeness and that all those affiliated with the hospital accept this as a desirable goal. This desire for a degree of autonomy, buttressed by the deferred monetary incentives discussed in chapter 4, should provide enough "carrots" to keep the system at the cutting edge of technological change and economic efficiency.

Any attempt here to elucidate and amplify this proposal would, I fear, only serve to confuse the issues. It should be recognized that the proposals presented are tentative guides to experimentation, that they are in the nature of transitional mechanisms and interim forms, and that no predetermined pattern is yet visualized. If in the longer view rational evaluation proves them inoperable and they are replaced by more cogent proposals the present consideration of them now will still have served its purpose.

Some 40 years ago the well-known economist, Walton H. Hamilton, in a statement appended to the Final Report of the Committee on the Costs of Medical Care observed that,

> . . . [T]he technology of medicine may be well developed, but the art of its organization is still in its infancy. We need to experiment, to find out new devices and procedures, and to combine them in organizations which may be vastly superior to anything which as yet we have tried.[1]

The present study, while it has neither described nor evaluated the changes in medical organization over four decades, would, I am afraid, appear to Hamilton as déjà vu. Another 40 years of the kind of change that has taken place during the preceding 40 will bring us into the twenty-first century with a system of health care unequal to the task at the beginning of the twentieth.

What the present work has attempted to do has been to look at hospitals that are at the core of the health system alternately through micro- and macroeconomic lenses. Our aim has been to bring into focus economic factors influencing the kind of health care that hospitals are actually delivering and to indicate how public policy might be applied at nodal points to elevate existing to higher levels of care, i.e. health services that are qualitatively superior, more accessible, and produced with greater efficiency.

It is evident that this has not been an exercise in cost-benefit analysis. It has been designed rather to draw attention to larger problems in the economics of hospital care and to provide a rationale and framework for subsequent application of cost-benefit or other decision-guidance approaches to specific features of organizational alternatives.

Our microeconomic view has centered around the concept of the hospital as a firm with associated inputs and outputs. While noting the difference between the profitseeking firm and the dominant nongovernmental, nonprofit voluntary hospital, we nevertheless have been inclined to the view that the conventional economic analysis of the firm can shed a good deal of light on the operations of the contemporary hospital. In particular, while the "firm" itself is "nonprofit," utilizing customary economic incentives for its employees should be increasingly relied upon to achieve efficiency.

We have examined the hospital's production function, i.e. the relationship between inputs and outputs, by bringing costs into our viewing field. The effect of supply-demand interrelations on hospital output, or occupancy rate, have been considered along with further discussion of the nature of hospital output and productivity. This led us into more refined definitions of input and output and of the calculation of what appear to us to be new measures of hospital output and productivity.

Given our findings, generally corroborative of other studies in this area, of relative inefficiency, we proceeded to focus on the potentials for and some techniques of intrahospital efficiency. Emphasis was placed on physical and functional reorganization as well as on the use of reimbursement as a tool for change. Our macroeconomic lens focused on systemic, i.e. interhospital problems. Finally, we advocated a policy of governmental supervision—not ownership and control—utilizing a public utility rate-setting mechanism combined with a federal health system modelled after the Federal Reserve System for over-all organizational coordination and direction.

The foregoing is a succinct summary of the topics treated above and of some of the conclusions reached. Aside from chapter 3, which hopefully presented a novel approach to hospital output and productivity, we have not undertaken any detailed empirical investigations of the analytical propositions discussed; the author has obviously drawn freely from the work of others in this regard. It is hoped that others will be moved to explore further and to refine some of the crude propositions regarding hospital economics that have been advanced here. Again, since we are dealing with an area that borders on organizational theory the need for interdisciplinary work in the health area is a particularly urgent one. It would be a source of great pleasure to the author if what was written here might serve to narrow the communications gaps that now exist and threaten to widen among the several social sciences concerned with health care. We can all of us, I think, agree with Ray Lyman Wilbur's dictum that, "The quality of medical care is an index of a civilization."[2] To raise that index should be a common goal that can and should be pursued by a pooling of disciplines, interests, and talents.

CHAPTER 1
   1. Research and Statistics Note, U.S. Department of Health,
       Education and Welfare, Social Security Administration,
       March 23, 1971, Table 1.1. See also, "Report to the
       President on Medical Care Prices," Washington, 1967.
   2. See E. Ginzberg, D. Hiestand, and B. Reubens, The
       Pluralistic Economy (New York: McGraw-Hill, 1965).
   3. Joseph P. Newhouse, "Toward a Theory of Nonprofit
       Institutions: An Economic Model of a Hospital,"
       American Economic Review, Vol. LX, No. 1, March
       1970, p. 64.
   4. For Comprehensive and incisive analyses of the role of the
       hospital see: Michael M. Davis, Medical Care for
       Tomorrow (New York: Harper, 1955); Herman M. and
       Anne Somers, Doctors, Patients and Health Insurance
       (Washington, D.C.: The Brookings Institution, 1961),
       especially Chapter X; Herbert E. Klarman, The Econom-
       ics of Health (New York: Columbia University Press,
       1965), Chapter V; H. M. and A. R. Somers, Medicare
       and the Hospitals (Washington, D.C.: The Brookings
       Institution, 1967), Chapter III.
   5. John Kenneth Galbraith, The New Industrial State (Boston:
       Houghton Mifflin, 1967), Chapter VI.
   6. Hospitals, Guide Issue, Part Two, August 1, 1970, p. 462.
   7. Edward M. Kaitz, Pricing Policy and Cost Behavior in the
       Hospital Industry (New York: Praeger Publishers,
       1968), p. 95.
   8. Joseph P. Newhouse, op. cit., p. 64.
   9. O. E. Williamson, "A Model of Rational Managerial
       Behavior" a chapter in A Behavioral Theory of the Firm
       by Richard M. Cyert and James G. March (Englewood
       Cliffs, N.J.: Prentice Hall, 1963), p. 241.
   10. Cyert and March, Ibid., p. 27.
   11. Williamson, op. cit., p. 278.
   12. J. K. Galbraith, op. cit., p. 354.

CHAPTER 2
   1. Seymour E. Harris, "Impact of Health Care Services and
       Programs on the Economy" in Methodology of Identifying,

Measuring and Evaluating Outcomes of Health Services Programs, Systems and Subsystems, Conference Series (Washington, D.C.: Department of Health, Education, and Welfare, Public Health Service, 1969).

2. Martin S. Feldstein, "The Rising Cost of Hospital Care," Discussion Paper Number 129, Harvard Institute of Economic Research (Cambridge, Mass.: Harvard University, August 1970), p. 95.

3. Ibid., p. 31.

4. Ibid., p. 97.

5. Ibid., pp. 87-88.

6. Ibid., Note 1, p. 87.

7. Ibid., p. 100.

8. Statement of Dr. John Freund Gillespie in "High Cost of Hospitalization," Hearings before the Subcommittee on Antitrust and Monopoly, Committee on the Judiciary, United States Senate, Ninety-First Congress, Second Session, February, April and May 1970, Part 1, p. 278.

9. Harry I. Greenfield, "Manpower Problems in the Allied Health Field," Journal of the American Medical Association, November 11, 1968, Vol. 206, p. 1,543.

10. Hospitals, Guide Issue, August 1, 1970, p. 463.

11. See, for example, the testimony of Gordon A. Friesen, in the "High Cost of Hospitalization," Hearings, loc. cit., pp. 545-571. Also, in Appendix F of "The Cost of the National Health Service in England and Wales" by Brian Abel-Smith and R. M. Titmuss (National Institute of Economic and Social Research, Cambridge, England, 1956), the authors report that the installation of new boilers was an important desire of hospital administrators and that, "nearly half [of the boilers] are estimated to yield returns of over 20 percent in running costs." Overall, in the cost-saving schemes reviewed by the authors involving a capital expenditure of 300,000 the annual saving in running costs would be about 70,000, indicating that the total capital expenditure would be recouped in only four years, p. 134.

12. Feldstein, op. cit., p. 3 (n. 1).

13. Martin S. Feldstein, Economic Analysis for Health Service Efficiency (Amsterdam: North Holland Publishing Company, 1967), p. 86.

14. See the lucid discussion of these points by Paul J. Feldstein in "Reimbursement Incentives for Hospital and Medical Care," Social Security Administration, Office of Research and Statistics, Research Report No. 26, March, 1968, p. 20 et. seq.

CHAPTER 3

1. Although related to the foregoing, the matter of the treatment of health expenditure data in our national product
   and income accounts is beyond the scope of this study.
   It might perhaps be mentioned in passing that the present
   writer has argued for the deduction of health expenditures
   from the GNP as human capital consumption allowances
   (depreciation) in the national accounts in "Medical Care
   in the United States: An Economic Work-up," presented
   to the Annual Meeting of the American Association for the
   Advancement of Science, December 26, 1965, in Cleveland,
   Ohio (unpublished).

2. See, for example, the paper by J. Douglas Colman, "An
   Analysis fo the Components of Rising Hospital Costs,"
   presented to the National Conference on Medical Costs,
   June 27, 1967, Washington, D.C., p. 6.

3. Comment by Martin S. Feldstein in, "Production and Productivity in the Service Industries," Victor R. Fuchs, ed.
   Studies in Income and Wealth, No. 34, National Bureau
   of Economic Research Inc., No. 7 (New York: Columbia
   University Press, 1969), p. 145 (n. 3).

4. Herbert E. Klarman, "The Increased Cost of Hospital Care,"
   chapter in the Economics of Health and Medical Care,
   S. J. Axelrod (ed.) (Ann Arbor: University of Michigan
   Press, 1964).

5. Herman M. Somers and Anne R. Somers, Medicare and the
   Hospitals, Brookings Studies in Social Economics
   (Washington, D.C.:   The Brookings Institution, 1967), p.77.

6. Martin S. Feldstein, "The Rising Cost of Hospital Care,"
   Harvard Institute of Economic Research, Cambridge,
   Mass., Discussion Paper Number 129, August, 1970, p. 25.

7. Ibid., p. 95.

8. Most recently in "High Cost of Hospitalization," Hearings
   before the Subcommittee on Antitrust and Monopoly of
   the Committee on the Judiciary, United States Senate,
   Ninety-first Congress, Second Session, Parts 1 and 2,
   1970 and 1971.

9. Harvey Leibenstein, "Allocative Efficiency vs. X Efficiency,"
   American Economic Review, June 1966, p. 398.

10. L. Vann Seawell, "Hospital Accounting and Financial Manage-
    ment" (Berwyn, Illinois: Physicians Record Company,
    1964), p. 405.

11. Ibid., p. 8.

12. Ibid., p. 378.

13. Ibid., p. 423.
14. Ibid., p. 431.
15. John H. Hayes, "Factors Affecting the Costs of Hospital
        Care," Vol. I of Financing Hospital Care in the United
        States (New York: The Blakiston Company, 1954), p. 76.
16. Hospitals, Guide Issue, August 1, 1969, Part Two, p. 466.
17. See Hospitals, Guide Issue, August 1, 1970, p. 468.
18. Ibid., p. 467.
19. Personal communication from James Ingram, Vice President,
        Associated Hospital Service of New York, to the author.
20. Irving Leveson, "Inflation and Quality in Public Programs,"
        Discussion Paper (mimeograph), New York City Planning
        Commission, December, 1970, p. 6.
21. For additional examples, see Table 3, "Percentage of
        Community Hospitals Reporting Services and Facilities
        by Hospital Size, 1968," Hospitals, Guide Issue, August 1,
        1969, p. 466.
22. Hospitals, Guide Issue, August 1, 1969, p. 468.
23. For a good general overview of these problems see Tech-
        nology and Manpower in the Health Service Industry, 1965-
        1975, U.S. Department of Labor, Manpower Research
        Bulletin, No. 14, May 1967, especially Appendix B-2,
        pp. 89-93.
24. Zvi Griliches, "Notes on the Measurement of Price and
        Quality Changes," Studies in Income and Wealth, Vol.
        28 (New York: National Bureau of Economic
        Research, 1964).

CHAPTER 4
1. Harvey Leibenstein, "Allocative Efficiency vs. X Efficiency."
        American Economic Review, June 1966, p. 408.
2. Ibid., p. 399.
3. Harry I. Greenfield, "Manpower Problems in the Allied
        Health Field," Journal of the American Medical Associa-
        tion, November 11, 1968, Vol. 206, p. 1,543.
4. Ibid., p. 1,543.
5. "High Cost of Hospitalization," Hearings before the Sub-
        committee on Antitrust and Monopoly of the Committee
        on the Judiciary, United States Senate, Ninety-first
        Congress, Second Session (1970), Part One, p. 70.
6. "Lowering the Cost of Medical Treatment (Strasbourg,
        France: Council of Europe. European Public Health
        Committee, March 1969), pp. 27 and 28.

7. Harry I. Greenfield, _Manpower and the Growth of Producer Services_ (New York: Columbia University Press, 1966), pp. 38-40.

8. "Management Engineering for Hospitals," American Hospital Association, Chicago, Illinois, 1970, p. 1. See also H. E. Smalley and J. R. Freeman, eds., _Hospital Industrial Engineering_ (New York: N. M. Reinhold Publishing Corp., 1966); U.S. Department of Labor, _Technology and Manpower in the Health Service Industry_, _Manpower Research Bulletin_, No. 14 (1967); "Operations Research in Hospitals," _Annals of the New York Academy of Sciences_, May 22, 1963.

9. Cited in "High Cost of Hospitalization," _op. cit._, p. 511.

10. Edward M. Kaitz, _Pricing Policy and Cost Behavior in the Hospital Industry_ (New York: Praeger Publishers, 1968) passim.

11. Ibid., p. v.

12. "High Cost of Hospitalization," _loc. cit._, Part 2, p. 71.

13. Kaitz, _op. cit._, pp. 51-2.

14. Ibid., p. 62.

15. Ibid., p. 68.

16. Ibid., p. 86.

17. Associated Hospital Service of New York, "Member Hospital Reimbursement Formula," December 31, 1969. See also "Principles of Reimbursement for Provider Costs and for Services by Hospital-Based Physicians," Regulations of the U.S. Department of Health, Education and Welfare (Reprint Date 2-70).

18. Ibid., pp. iii and iv; see also Chapter 957 of the Laws of New York, 1969, and Part 86 of the Administrative Rules and Regulations of the [New York] State Commissioner of Health, July 1, 1970.

19. Ibid., p. 1.

20. Letter to the author from the Division of Health Economics of the State of New York Department of Health, dated April 6, 1971.

21. _The New York Times_, September 13, 1971.

22. Eleanor G. Gilpatrick and Paul K. Corlins, _The Occupational Structure of New York City Municipal Hospitals_ (New York: Praeger Publishers, 1970), p. 6.

23. J. J. Jehring, "Increasing Productivity in Hospitals," Center for the Study of Productivity Motivation, Graduate School of Business, The University of Wisconsin (Madison, Wisconsin, 1966), p. 4.

24. Ibid., p. 57.
25. Ibid., p. 61.
26. John Schiel, "Subsystem Incentives at Baptist Hospital,
    Pensacola, Florida" in Incentive Management for Hospitals—
    Proceedings of a Conference, June 5-6, 1968. University
    of Wisconsin, J. J. Jehring et al. (Washington, D.C.:
    Clearinghouse for Federal Scientific and Technical
    Information, U.S. Department of Commerce, September
    1969), p. 41.
27. Ibid., p. 44.

CHAPTER 5
1. Anne R. Somers, Hospital Regulation: The Dilemma of
   Public Policy. Industrial Relations Section, Princeton
   University (Princeton, N.J.: Princeton University Press,
   1969), Research Report Series No. 112, p. 133.
2. David D. Rutstein, The Coming Revolution in Medicine
   (Cambridge: M.I.T. Press, 1967), p. 76.
3. "Lowering the Cost of Medical Treatment, "Strasbourg,
   France: Council of Europe, European Public Health
   Committee, March 1969), p. 24.
4. Ibid., pp. 32-33.
5. The New York Times, September 20, 1971.
6. Mark Blumberg, "Shared Services for Hospitals" (Chicago:
   American Hospital Association, 1966), p. 20. See also
   the reports of merger and sharing activities in David
   B. Starkweather and Shirley J. Taylor, "Health Facility
   Combinations and Mergers: An Annotated Bibliography"
   (Chicago: American College of Hospital Administrators,
   February 1970).
7. Blumberg, Ibid., pp. 16, 22.
8. Cecil G. Sheps, "Trends in Hospital Care" Inquiry, Vol.
   VIII, No. 1, March 1971, p. 27.
9. Report of the New York Governor's Committee on Hospital
   Costs New York, December 15, 1965, p. 90.
10. Ibid., p. 23.
11. Walter J. McNerney and Donald C. Riedel, "Regionalization
    and Rural Health Care," Michigan University, Bureau of
    Hospital Administration, Research Series No. 2 (Ann
    Arbor: University of Michigan, 1962), p. 4.
12. Ibid,, Forward.
13. "Report of the Task Force on Medicaid and Related Pro-
    grams" Washington, D.C.: U.S. Department of Health,
    Education and Welfare, June 29, 1970, pp. 4-5.

14. Ibid., p. 26. See also Herman M. and Anne R. Somers, Medicare and the Hospitals (Washington, D.C.: The Brookings Institution, 1967), passim.

15. Anne R. Somers, op. cit., p. 203.

16. Ibid., pp. 204-08.

17. Clair Wilcox, Public Policies Toward Business (Richard D. Irwin, Inc., Third Edition, 1966), p. 287.

18. Anne R. Somers, op. cit., p. 207.

19. Task Force, op. cit., p. 28.

20. Ibid., pp. 169-70.

21. "Government Investment in Health Care," Scientific American, April 1971, p. 25.

22. Anne R. Somers, op. cit., pp. 169-70.

23. Anne R. Somers, "Health Care in Transition: Directions for the Future" (Chicago: Hospital Research and Educational Trust, 1971), p. 108.

24. Ibid., p. 109. The counterpart within a single hospital of community averaging is the presently extremely limited practice of reimbursement by inclusive rates. In place of an itemized bill that lists all of the ancillary services separately the patient receives an average bill based on hospital-wide costs and usage. See "Reimbursing Hospitals on Inclusive Rates," The Boston Consulting Group, Boston, Mass., under contract with the National Center for Health Services Research and Development, 1970.

CHAPTER 6

1. Medical Care for the American People, The Final Report of the Committee on the Costs of Medical Care, adopted in Washington, D.C., October 31, 1932 (Reprinted 1970 by U.S. Department of Health, Education and Welfare, Public Health Service), p. 198.

2. Ibid., Introduction, p. xix.

HARRY I. GREENFIELD is Professor of Economics at Queens College of the City University of New York and Senior Research Associate at the Center For Policy Research Inc.

Dr. Greenfield has published in the field of general economics as well as in the economics of health. Two previous books are: Manpower and the Growth of Producer Services and Allied Health Manpower: Trends and Prospects, both by Columbia University Press. His articles and reviews have appeared in: Journal of the American Medical Association; American Journal of Public Health; Bulletin of the New York Academy of Medicine; Monthly Labor Review; Quarterly Review of Economics and Business; The Financial Analysts Journal; The Commercial and Financial Chronicle; and Computers and Automation.

Dr. Greenfield holds a B.S.S. from City College of the City University of New York and an M.A. and Ph.D. from Columbia University.

COAL MINE HEALTH AND SAFETY:
The Case of West Virginia

J. Davitt McAteer

A COST-EFFECTIVENESS STUDY OF CLINICAL METHODS OF
BIRTH CONTROL:
With Special Reference to Puerto Rico

William J. Kelly

DOCTORS IN POLITICS:
The Political Life of the Japan Medical Association

William E. Steslicke

MANPOWER SUBSTITUTION IN THE HOSPITAL INDUSTRY:
A Study of New York City Voluntary and Municipal Systems

Myron D. Fottler

MEDICAL CARE AT PUBLIC EXPENSE:
A Study in Applied Welfare Economics

Mark V. Pauly

PARAPROFESSIONALS AND THEIR PERFORMANCE:
A Survey of Education, Health, and Social Service Programs

Alan Gartner

PLANNED CHANGE IN THE HOSPITAL:
Case Studies of Organizational Innovations

Rodney M. Coe

THE POLITICS OF HEALTH CARE:
Nine Case Studies of Innovative Planning in New York City

Herbert Harvey Hyman